NEUROMOTOR MECHANISMS IN HUMAN COMMUNICATION

OXFORD PSYCHOLOGY SERIES

1. *The neuropsychology of anxiety: an enquiry into the functions of the septohippocampal system*
   Jeffrey A. Gray
2. *Elements of episodic memory*
   Endel Tulving
3. *Conditioning and associative learning*
   N. J. Mackintosh
4. *Visual masking: an integrative approach*
   Bruno G. Breitmeyer
5. *The musical mind: the cognitive psychology of music*
   John Sloboda
6. *Elements of psychophysical theory*
   J.-C. Falmagne
7. *Animal intelligence*
   Edited by L. Weiskrantz
8. *Response times: their role in inferring elementary mental organization*
   R. Duncan Luce
9. *Mental representations: a dual coding approach*
   Allan Paivio
10. *Memory, imprinting, and the brain*
    Gabriel Horn
11. *Working memory*
    Alan Baddeley
12. *Blindsight: a case study and implications*
    L. Weiskrantz
13. *Profile analysis*
    D. M. Green
14. *Spatial vision*
    R. L. DeValois and K. K. DeValois
15. *The neural and behavioural organization of goal-directed movements*
    Marc Jeannerod
16. *Visual pattern analyzers*
    Norma V. Graham
17. *Cognitive foundations of musical pitch analysis*
    C. L. Krumhansl
18. *Perceptual and associative learning*
    G. Hall
19. *Implicit learning and tacit knowledge: an essay on the cognitive unconscious*
    Arthur S. Reber
20. *Neuromotor mechanisms in human communication*
    Doreen Kimura

Neuromotor Mechanisms in Human Communication

Doreen Kimura
Department of Psychology
The University of Western Ontario

OXFORD PSYCHOLOGY SERIES
NO. 20

New York Oxford
OXFORD UNIVERSITY PRESS · CLARENDON PRESS
1993

Oxford University Press

Oxford New York Toronto
Delhi Bombay Calcutta Madras Karachi
Kuala Lumpur Singapore Hong Kong Tokyo
Nairobi Dar es Salaam Cape Town
Melbourne Auckland
and associated companies in
Berlin Ibadan

Published by Oxford University Press, Inc.,
200 Madison Avenue, New York, New York 10016

Oxford is a registered trade mark of Oxford University Press

Library of Congress Cataloging in Publication Data
Kimura, Doreen.
Neuromotor mechanisms in human communication / Doreen Kimura.
p. cm.—(Oxford psychology series ; no. 20)
Includes bibliographical references and index.
ISBN 0-19-505492-X
1. Neurolinguistics. 2. Psycholinguistics. 3. Communicative disorders—Pathophysiology. 4. Efferent pathways. I. Title. II. Series.
[*DNLM: 1. Brain—physiology. 2. Communication. 3. Psychomotor Performance—physiology.* WL 300 K485n]
QP399.K56 1993
153.6—dc20
DNLM/DLC
for Library of Congress
92-49194

9 8 7 6 5 4 3 2 1

Printed in the United States of America
on acid-free paper

This monograph is dedicated to
the late Donald Olding Hebb and to Brenda Milner
who introduced me to neuropsychology

Acknowledgments

I am grateful first of all to Hugo Liepmann whose originality of thought and whose inventiveness in the behavior-based analysis of apraxia is still a model for Neuropsychology to emulate. Liepmann might well be considered the first *behavioral* neuroscientist.

I want especially to thank Neil Watson and Bryan Kolb for their patience in reading the entire manuscript and providing me with much valuable advice about revisions. Two anonymous reviewers chosen by Oxford University Press also made very helpful comments. Graduate students in Psychobiology/Neuropsychology at the University of Western Ontario read some of the chapters and provided useful criticism.

The data could not have been collected without the support of the faculty in the departments of Clinical Neurological Sciences and in Rehabilitation Medicine. I am particularly grateful to Dr. H. J. M. Barnett for his invaluable assistance in establishing a research base initially at University Hospital. I want also to acknowledge the patients who gave their time and effort to the project.

Much of the data analysis was done by Neil Watson, or is based on the computerized database he established, along with Rob Faust and Wilda Davidson. I had help with figures and tables from Corinne Toussaint, Michael Carson, Barbara Peck, and Jane Hammingh.

The research on which this monograph is based spanned almost 20 years. It was supported by grants from the Medical Research Council and the Natural Sciences and Engineering Research Council, Ottawa, Canada.

D.K.
University of Western Ontario
London, Ontario, Canada

August 1992

Contents

NEUROMOTOR MECHANISMS IN HUMAN COMMUNICATION

1. Introduction

The term "communication" refers to a variety of behaviors, including the interactions of living organisms with inanimate objects such as computers. The term is used here in a narrower sense, to refer to the behaviors by which one member of a species conveys information to another member of the species; the focus will be on human communication systems, though within a comparative/evolutionary framework. Our information about the neural systems underlying human communication has come largely from the study of disruptions in speech which are experienced by the individual who has suffered damage to the central nervous system. In the past, such disorders, called "aphasias" and usually resulting from damage to the left cerebral hemisphere, have nearly always been attributed to an underlying disorder of *language*. Thus aphasic disorders have been studied primarily with regard to linguistic concepts like phoneme, morpheme, semantics, syntactics, and so forth, which presuppose that speech is organized and disorganized in the brain according to such categories.

One consequence of this approach is the expectation that movements generated during speaking will be controlled by neural systems separate from those involved in nonspeech functions. That is, linguistic movements are assumed to be generated by a special system in the brain, and nonlinguistic movements of the same musculature are not expected to be affected in aphasic disorders. This might be a reasonable expectation if all aphasias were considered to be solely linguistic disorders, and if language systems were entirely superordinate to their motor control and expression. That, in fact, is how most neurolinguists view language. The exception allowed within this schema is a type of aphasia called "Broca's aphasia," which is assumed to be primarily a *motor* speech disorder, in contrast to other types of aphasia. According to such conceptualizations, Broca's aphasia reflects the interface between "language" and the endpoint motor control systems of speech. Paradoxically, the existence of such a severe speech productionproblem after left-hemisphere damage appears to have encouraged the view that the remaining speech systems (reflected in other kinds of aphasia) are involved primarily in a linguistic code, rather than in other levels of motor control.

This book, in contrast, will suggest an approach to the neural basis of communication which emphasizes behavioral analysis, rather than linguistic or cognitive processes. Very little of the literature on the neuropsychology of speech actually deals with the behavior of *speaking*. Much of it relates to the semantic and syntactic frameworks within which speech is presumed to be organized. While undeniably important, these may not be the only or even the primary features affected in aphasia, and dependent on the left hemisphere.

To reiterate, there are two common assumptions about the neural mechanisms of human communication which are related, and whose validity will be questioned: (1) that the critical role of the left hemisphere in communication is based on a specialization for linguistic/semantic function, and (2) that language behavior is organized quite separately from nonlanguage behaviors in the brain.

What will be proposed instead is that human communication has, during the course of evolution, become intrinsically bound to the various motor programming systems that control the relevant musculature. The characteristics of such motor programming systems are presumed to have been determined by a variety of constraints, only one of which is the use of these systems for communication. Thus, the presumption will be that our communication systems have been shaped in part by the characteristics of certain motor systems. This view shifts the emphasis from speech per se as the focus of study, to the neural mechanisms of movement selection, manual as well as vocal. The early freeing of the arms from locomotor function in hominids and the strong propensity for humans to employ a manual system of communication when the auditory–vocal system is defective suggest that manual systems of communication might have evolved early in hominid history (Hewes, 1973). This may also be reflected in the relative ease with which the great apes can be taught a manual as compared to a vocal language. Knowing something about the neural mechanisms controlling arm and hand movements may thus elucidate the characteristics of human communication systems in general.

Communication in the great apes

Continuity of modern human communication systems with those of other primate species, as well as with early hominids, will be assumed. The question whether nonhuman primates possess the capacity for *language* will of course be answered by how that term is defined. Behaviorally, we may define language as a system of self-generated movements, composed of definable units, which can arbitrarily represent some object, event, or intention on the part of the mover (Kimura, 1979). It is obvious that we can elaborate definitions of language in such a way that only human beings could be said to be capable of it. However, we might similarly define language in such a way that only chimpanzees are seen to be capable of it. For example, Menzel (1973) has shown that chimpanzees can communicate to each other the location and nature of food without gestures or vocalizations, apparently by using some type of whole-body communication not decodable by human experimenters. Whenever we compare different species, we will find behaviors that are unique in the sense of being idiosyncratic. The strategy of the extreme humanist, when faced with the sometimes amazing achievements of the great apes in problem solving or communication, is to respond with "Yes, perhaps they can do this, but not that, which only humans can do." This approach is fruitful only when it helps to define a valid dimension along which behavior can be scaled.

A list compiled by Hockett (1960) of the characteristics of animal communication systems still serves as a useful framework for discussion. Human language is said to have a number of characteristics which are only partly, or not at all, shared by nonhuman communication systems. Some of the more significant are:

semanticity—the ability to use a sign or symbol to stand for a referent (for example, a name which refers to an object);
arbitrariness—the sign does not necessarily resemble its referent, especially true of speech, where names do not usually resemble their referents;
displacement—the ability to refer to things or events not present;
productivity—the capacity to generate new, not previously used signs or sign combinations;
traditional transmission—learned from conspecifics, a characteristic which follows from arbitrariness;
duality of patterning—the fact that a particular morpheme (or its equivalent) may mean different things in different combinations, a feature which has also been called recombinance (for example, "dog" has different significance in "doghouse" and "dogdays").
Finally, most people would also add *syntax*—the order of signs in an utterance can change the meaning of the utterance, as in "She dislikes burning the leaves" and "She dislikes the burning leaves."

Since human communication typically employs the vocal musculature, it seemed natural for scientists interested in studying nonhuman primates to focus on their ability to use speech. This anthropomorphic approach was sometimes carried to extremes, such as the case in which a chimpanzee was reared in a human family with a child (see Table 1). Many, as it turns out, fruitless hours were spent attempting to teach the unfortunate chimp human speech sounds. The pinnacle of success among such home-reared chimps was Viki, who learned to utter about four intelligible words, though she apparently understood about 50 others (Hayes, 1951). Since this was the result of several years of

Table 1.1 Human speech in the great apes

Author	Training	Results
Witmer, 1909	yes	"mama" (unvoiced vowel)
Furness, 1916*	yes	"papa" "cup"
Kellogg, 1932	no	—
Kohts, 1935	no	—
Hayes, 1951	yes ($6\frac{1}{2}$ years)	"mama" "papa" "cup" "up"? (single hoarse vowel for all)

Source: After Kellogg, 1968.
* An orangutan; all others are chimpanzees.

intensive training, it seemed to indicate that the chimpanzee was hopelessly incapable of learning a language. Such incapacity was generally attributed to limitations of brain organizations—that is, that some critical requirements of linguistic capacity were simply absent.

Philip Lieberman, however, suggested that the chimpanzee's vocal tract is so different from human's that it is not capable of forming human speech sounds (Lieberman, 1975). This would of course be a severe limitation, quite apart from any differences between humans and apes in neural control mechanisms. That there may also be other limitations to the chimpanzee's control of vocalization is suggested by Yerkes and Learned's (1925) unsuccessful attempt to condition spontaneous vocalizations. Jürgens (1979) has reported failure to condition specific vocalizations in monkeys also, though they can be trained to emit or suppress vocalizations (Jürgens, 1989*a*). The fact that no vocalizations of any kind can be elicited in monkeys by neocortical stimulation (Robinson, 1967), whereas crude vowel-like sounds can be elicited in humans (Penfield & Roberts, 1959), suggests that voicing may be under cortical control only in humans. In nonhuman primates, vocalization appears to be closely tied to the animal's specific motivational state.

Kellogg (1968), one of those psychologists who adopted a chimpanzee and attempted to teach it speech, remarked in retrospect that he ought to have considered using manual gestures instead, since their chimpanzee, Gua, often attempted to use such gestures. These attempts were naturally steadfastly ignored by her speech-oriented trainers. The fact that chimpanzees use brachial and whole-body gestures in the wild, according to Goodall (1971), also indicates that manual gestures comprise a much more appropriate vehicle for the study of symbolic capacity in the great apes than does vocalization.

The first successful attempt to teach a manual language to a chimpanzee was made by Gardner and Gardner (1969), with their now-famous pupil Washoe. Training took place in very much the same circumstances as that in which the human child learns speech—during everyday activities such as eating, dressing, toilet training, and play. Washoe acquired over 100 signs ultimately, and this record of achievement has been exceeded by other chimpanzees subsequently trained by the Gardners and by their collaborator and student, Roger Fouts. They established many parallels between the way the chimps learn to sign and the signing of young children, including the kinds of mistakes made by both (Gardner & Gardner, 1971). Later a manual sign language was also successfully taught to a gorilla (Patterson, 1978).

Such signing behaviors in apes constitute a rough parallel to the way we use language. Consider the following characteristics:

(1) *Semanticity*—there is no doubt that the chimpanzee and gorilla have the ability to use a sign or symbol to stand for a referent. The simple fact of their signing vocabulary attests to this, and further evidence of the nonstereotypical use of such signs suggests that these are not simply responses fixed to certain stimulus conditions.

(2) *Arbitrariness*—although many signs acquired by the great apes are iconic (e.g., toothbrush, drink), many more are not (e.g., dirty, more).

(3) *Displacement*—there have been innumerable instances of the use of a sign in the absence of the referent, as well as in the absence of immediate context.

(4) *Productivity*—this is more problematic, because productivity would arise frequently only when there is a great deal of spontaneous signing with other conspecifics. It is quite clear that chimps and gorillas do not spend a lot of time signing to each other, at least not using identifiable manual gestures. Nevertheless, a number of unequivocal instances of the generation of new composites of signs have been reported (Fouts, 1973; Patterson, 1978).

(5) *Transmission to other conspecifics*—there is some evidence that chimpanzees have learned a significant number of signs without human intervention.

The conclusion that the great apes use sign language in qualitatively the same way that native human signers do has been much criticized (Seidenberg & Petitto, 1978; Terrace, 1985). Some of these criticisms have focused on the lack of precision of the gestures, the fact that they are often employed in a noncommunicative situation, and the relatively sparse use of them for spontaneous communication with conspecifics. Such comments ignore the fact that the chimpanzee musculature is not precisely like our own, and that chimps after all do not need a manual system of communication to interact with each other, since they possess a successful facial and whole-body system. Therefore, we would not expect them to employ what is essentially an extremely foreign language except under very constrained circumstances. Moreover, young human infants learning signs (and speech) intersperse signing with non-communicative "babbling," and yet we do not discount such expressions as nonlanguage. Underlying much of the criticism from the scientific sign-language community is the implication that if a chimpanzee can learn a manual sign language, however crudely, but not a vocal language, the sign language will appear to be degraded. (This is of course nonsensical and irrelevant.)

However, the critical questions are surely not whether the great apes have demonstrated human levels of expertise, subtlety, and productivity in signing. Of course they have not, and they almost certainly will never do so. No more would human beings be able to learn to hoot and stamp in an alarming situation exactly as a chimpanzee does. The crux of the significance of the work of the Gardners, Fouts, and Patterson is that the great apes *can* employ, at the very least, a rudimentary manual sign language when constrained to do so, *demonstrating that the capacity is there to be selected, as it appears to have been in humans.*

These studies have also told us that the symbolic or semantic capabilities of the great apes may be well above anything that has previously been apparent to human observers. These capabilities have been further elaborated by Premack (1971), employing a procedure in which meaningless objects are used to represent real objects or events. A large array of such object labels is readily learned by the chimpanzee, and in this situation she exhibits a high level of semanticity. (As in most of the great-ape language studies, Premack's subject is female.) Not only could she acquire object names, but also concepts like "name of," "negatives," and so on. One should say, rather, that this procedure allowed us to *see* the level of semanticity; it was simply not adequately probed before. Hewes' (1977) comment is pertinent: "the successes being achieved by chimpanzee language-learners must rest on the already existing ability of these animals to understand the world in much the same way that we do."

Communication in early hominids

If it is difficult to establish the intellectual characteristics of animals like the great apes, which still exist, it is obviously even more difficult to do so for species now extinct, such as early forms of human beings. The only tangible evidence is structural or physical—the kinds of skeletons they possessed, and the artifacts they left. These are important clues, but often they only tantalize us with the possible, rather than telling us what actually occurred. The limitation of inferences from artifacts, for example, is indicated by the popular and probably correct assumption that very early man used clubs made of tree limbs or bones. There is, however, no direct physical evidence for this, because unshaped pieces of wood or bone do not permit inferences about their use. In addition, because wood seldom leaves a fossil trace, shaped wooden artifacts would be absent from the fossil record.

Considering first the vocal system of communication, what can we deduce about the complexity of speech in early hominids? The suggestion that the chimpanzee does not have the requisite vocal tract for generating human speech sounds has already been noted (Lieberman, 1975). Studying the reconstructions of supralaryngeal vocal tracts from early hominids, Lieberman has concluded that the modern human vocal tract appeared less than half a million years ago. It was not present in *Australopithecus*, *Homo habilis*, nor, according to Lieberman, in so recent a hominid as Neanderthal man (see Table 1.2). Figure 1.1 illustrates a simple version of the supralaryngeal vocal tract in a modern adult human, a human infant, and in *Australopithecus*. The adult human is capable of making all of the complex sounds we employ, but the infant is not. According to Lieberman, the right-angled shape of the adult human vocal tract is a prerequisite for the production of the three critical vowels (as in "hod," "heed," and "who'd"), which are an essential feature of modern human speech. Thus while vocal sounds could certainly be made without this right-angled tract, the complexity of speech would be limited, with the stop consonants especially affected. If this view is correct, it would indicate that the evolution of complex speech was a rather late development, appearing long after the advent of upright walking and of complex tool use.

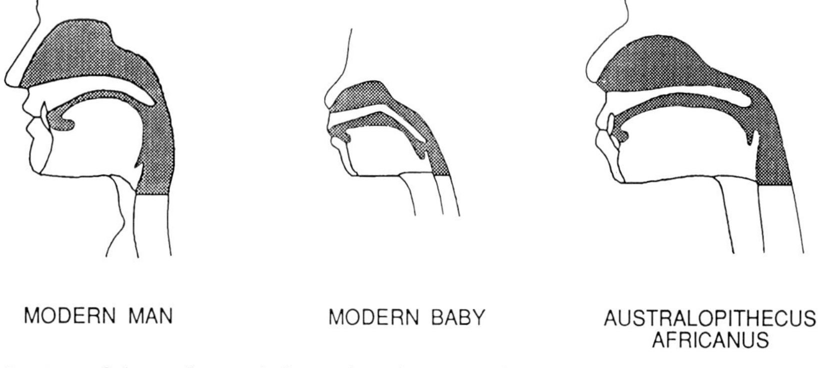

Fig. 1.1 Schematic variations in the supralaryngeal vocal tract. (After Lieberman, 1975.)

Table 1.2 A summary of hominid ancestors

Years before present	Species	Characteristics
8 million	*Ramapithecus*	Teeth have some similarity with hominids
4 million	*Australopithecus afarensis*	Completely upright walker; relatively small brain; teeth have some similarity to *H. sapiens* and to *A. africanus*
2.5 million	*Australopithecus africanus*	Upright walker; use of bones as clubs?; may have coexisted with *Homo habilis* and not be ancestral to *Homo erectus*
2 million	*Homo habilis*	Upright walker; tool user
1 million	*Homo erectus*	Abundant tool use; relatively large brain
$\frac{1}{2}$ million	*Homo sapiens*	Modern man

Source: After Johanson and Edey, 1981.

This does not mean that only a crude system of communication was available until recently. *Homo habilis*, over a million years ago, could not only use objects as tools but could shape tools as well. Thus, deliberately shaped tools usable as hand axes, chisels, scrapers, and so on, existed in association with *Homo habilis* sites (Leakey, 1979). The neural control of the manual and brachial musculature must have been extensive in order for such tool use and tool formation to occur. The fact that modern humans can readily learn a manual language, and that chimpanzees and gorillas can learn a manual system to a fairly high level, makes it probable that complex manual systems developed before complex vocal systems. It is probable, therefore, although it cannot be proven, that a manual system of communication was employed by early hominids; and that it was considerably more complex than the vocal system available at the same time (see Hewes, 1973, 1977). The degree of complexity and subtlety which are possible within a manual system of communication is outlined in Chapter 8 which discusses manual sign language.

Methods in studying the neurology of language

The history of investigation into the neural systems involved in speaking has largely been one of describing salient speech disorders in individual cases of brain damage. Delineating the extent and locus of the underlying neural pathology has been secondary, in the sense that where it is done at all, it has nearly always been with reference only to positive instances of particular aphasic syndromes. The alternative approach, studying the effects, or lack thereof, of a particular locus of pathology on speech, is almost nonexistent. Yet *knowledge of the frequency of both occurrence and nonoccurrence of particular aphasic symptoms is equally important to understanding the contribution of specific brain regions to speech* in normal persons. If we look only at the occurrence of positive symptoms, we may severely misjudge the generalizability of our findings, and we may miss important individual variation in brain organization.

A simple analogy may illustrate the problem. Imagine that in one year at a neurological hospital, 20 people suffer damage to a particular region of the brain, called area X. One of the researchers at this hospital is interested in the neural mechanisms underlying semantic categories, and therefore arranges to have all patients who appear to have intellectual problems at bedside testing referred. These patients are then given a test which requires them to label brands of beer, as well as a test requiring the labeling of brands of soft drinks. The researcher is especially interested in *dissociations* of categories, and so has a research assistant select for further investigation all patients who show a significant deficit in beer-labeling, relative to soft-drink-labeling ability. Four such patients are identified in the course of the year, and when the maps of their brain lesions are overlapped, they all have significant damage to area X. The researcher concludes that (1) there is a distinct functional system for the categorizing and labeling of beer, and (2) area X comprises such a system.

This example may seem a bit far-fetched, but it is unfortunately not unlike much of the neurological and neuropsychological case-history compilation research which is published, particularly in the field of aphasiology. What are some of the problems with this type of approach?

First, we are making inferences about the function of an anatomical system based on a minority of cases with damage to that system. What of the 16 additional patients with damage to area X? Presumably they show no such dissociation, and in fact were not even selected for further testing on the basis of the bedside assessment. Is it appropriate to conclude, on the basis of four out of 20 cases, that area X generally plays a critical role in beer-labeling but not soft-drink-labeling? Or is the finding merely an artifact of idiosyncratic background in these four people (they may be teetotallers)?

Second, without sampling a range of normal behaviors, we cannot be certain that beer-labeling is not slightly more difficult than soft-drink-labeling, and therefore that a number of patients with mild naming problems will score somewhat lower on the beer-labeling task. Even if we had normative data on the two tests, we might not detect small differences in difficulty level, because both tests are significantly easier for normal persons than they are for people who are somewhat disadvantaged intellectually by brain damage.

Third, the initial method of selection for testing is less than optimal, in that there might be other patients who have greater beer-labeling than soft-drink-labeling deficits, but they are never identified because they do not show deficits at bedside examination which were evident to the medical resident. For example, they may be severely impaired in all kinds of naming, and thus appear inappropriate for inclusion. Some of these patients may have lesions outside area X.

Fourth, this approach assumes that the extremes of a distribution ipso facto form a separate entity—that is, that those four people who are divergent in their beer-labeling are functionally different from the others, rather then representing just the extremes of a normal distribution. But we could make this kind of claim for almost any function, however trivial, for example, thumb size, or simple reaction time.

Fifth, dividing scores into two groups, by means of a "cutoff" score, may result in an artifactual dissociation. For example, a case is below the cutoff on one test, and above the cutoff on the other test, yet both scores might be near the mean of each distribution. Such arbitrary classification may oscure the real relationship between the tests. Cutoff scores necessarily exaggerate dissociations. (See Bates, Appelbaum, & Allard, 1991, for further discussion of the problems of dissociations in single cases.)

Sixth, one or both of the tests used may be insufficiently reliable, or the scores may be unreliable because the patient's pathology is in a fluctuating state. Thus, the dissociation between two functions could be an artifact of errors of measurement. Inferences made entirely on the basis of dissociations in individual cases need more convincing evidence of the reliability of each of the tests being compared than is true for group data, but this condition is rarely satisfied.

These are just some of the fallacies which may be detected, and which we should keep in mind, as we attempt to evaluate the findings from studies of this kind. This does not mean that we will never find out anything from studying the individual case, but it does mean that we must be very cautious in making general conclusions from individual cases. (For an in-depth consideration of some of these cautions, see Shallice, 1988.) Such generalizations become even more problematic when we realize that there are systematic individual variations in the way some functions are organized in the brain (see Chapters 9 and 10).

It may appear that famous cases in the literature like HM, the amnesic described by Scoville and Milner (1957), have provided an ideal prototype for the study of certain functional systems. But it should be remembered that HM was just one of several cases with extensive medial temporal resection, all of whom had symptoms very similar to his. Had he been very divergent from the other cases, it is problematic whether his amnestic pattern should have had the impact that it did on the neuropsychology of memory. Of course, individual cases may suggest ideas about how various psychological functions are mediated in the brain, which may then be systematically investigated in additional less selected series of cases.

The present investigation

This monograph will present findings from the study of patients with unilateral cerebral pathology. It differs from most other studies of this kind in that patients were not chosen or studied for particular symptomatology. Instead, we studied all patients who were well enough to undergo two to three hours of testing, and who agreed to take part in the investigation. The only criteria were the presumptive unilaterality of the lesion at the time of testing, and an age limit of 70 or less.

The focus of the investigation was the relationship between communicative and noncommunicative functions. In particular, we studied the ability to make a variety of oral and manual movements, and how these abilities related to speech function. The evidence from these studies suggests that the left hemisphere is predominant (in right-handers) for a wide range of behaviors in which motor selection is critical, regardless of their linguistic content. Its role in human language is argued to be secondary to such motor function. The early chapters will outline the pervasiveness of left-hemisphere motor control in both cortical and noncortical systems. The nature of the oral and manual programming vested in the left hemisphere will be elaborated, as well as its contribution to constructional ability and manual sign language. This will be contrasted with its relatively minor role in representation/semantic functions. Finally, systematic variation in brain organization, related to the sex and hand preference of the individual, will be reported. Exhaustive reviews of the literature will not be attempted, generally only enough background being given to enable the reader to see the context and relevance of the empirical findings.

Patients included in the study were seen over almost a 20-year time span, from the early seventies to 1990. The tests that were administered naturally changed over time, as data accumulated and generated new questions. Hence, the number of patients seen on any one test was smaller than the total sample. However, at any point in time, all patients were given all the tests in the current "battery," with the exception of the more intensive testing of speech functions in aphasic patients, compared to nonaphasics. Actual sample size will be given for each test as it is discussed. Details are given in the "Tests and Procedures" section which follows.

The patient sample

Lateralized sample

Over the first 10 years, all patients were seen at the local University Hospital, but in later years patients from two other hospitals were investigated as well. The final decision about lateralization of the lesion was typically made two to three months after the patient had been tested, when all diagnostic data were collected and appeared in the hospital chart. If at that time there was evidence of bilaterality of pathology, the data were not included.

In all, 314 patients with left-hemisphere pathology and 207 with right-hemisphere pathology were assessed. Most of these were cases of vascular accidents, predominantly strokes, a significant number were tumors, and the remainder were of mixed etiology, largely seizure cases. Table 1.3 gives characteristics of the sample. These patients are all right-handed, left-handers being dealt with separately in Chapter 9.

Diagnostic information for most patients was available from computed tomography scans. On vascular cases, angiography had also typically been performed, and on seizure cases EEGs were available. Where there was a significant mass effect or midline shift which could affect the other hemisphere, the patient was excluded from the unilateral category. In cases of doubt the radiologist was consulted for a final decision.

It is clear from Table 1.3 that males are encountered more frequently in our sample, particularly in those cases with vascular accidents, and that left-sided cases are more common than are right-sided cases, in

Table 1.3 The total patient sample

	Left lesions (314)		Right lesions (207)	
Pathology	Male[a] (200)	Female[b] (114)	Male[c] (115)	Female[d] (92)
Vascular	148 (74%)	67 (59%)	82 (71%)	65 (71%)
Tumor	41 (21%)	32 (28%)	25 (22%)	18 (20%)
Other	11 (6%)	15 (13%)	8 (7%)	9 (10%)

Mean ages (years): a, 52.8; b, 47.8; c, 51.2; d, 46.8.

Table 1.4 Patients with localized lesions within a hemisphere

	Left lesions (131)		Right lesions (88)	
Locus	Male	Female	Male	Female
Anterior	18	14	12	15
Central	13	10	13	9
Posterior	46	30	18	21

agreement with the literature in Caucasian samples (Marquardsen, 1969; Bogousslavsky, Van Melle, & Regli, 1988). The side of pathology in our sample differs between men and women for the vascular cases only ($\chi^2 = 6.42$, df $= 1$, $p < .02$). Thus, the distribution across left and right hemispheres is quite equal in women, but vascular accidents favor the left hemisphere in men. There does not appear to be any information in the literature concerning possible sex differences in hemisphere-of-lesion, though the Marquardsen study shows the same trend as our data. However, when considering more localized pathology (Table 1.4), there are no significant differences between men and women in left–right distribution, for any type of pathology, including vascular.

Localization within the hemisphere

Where feasible within lateralized groups, more precise localization of the lesion was attempted. The major classification was threefold:

(1) Anterior—pathology restricted to in front of the central (Rolandic) fissure and excluding any part of the temporal lobe.
(2) Posterior—lesion was behind the central fissure but might include the temporal lobe.
(3) Central—lesion involved primarily the pre- and/or postcentral gyrus.

Patients who had a significant hemiparesis *and* either a visual field defect or significantly raised two-point threshold on the contralateral side were excluded from further consideration for anterior or posterior localization. As in the case of lesion lateralization, where there was doubt the radiologist was consulted and his decision used for final localization. Localization was determined for a group of cases about once a year, and the neuropsychological data were not consulted in the process.

Data on the total sample of patients with localized pathology are presented in Table 1.4. Just over 40% of lateralized cases have localizable lesions, in each hemisphere. Over half of these have posterior lesions, the numbers in the anterior and central groups being relatively small. The larger numbers in the posterior-locus group made possible the further subdivision of this group into viable subgroups, for some tests, of temporal- or parietal-lobe lesions.

Tests and procedures

In the early years of our study, an intelligence test was administered to most patients, but in later years only certain subtests were administered, as described below. In addition, a variety of tests sampling the presence or absence of aphasia and apraxia (oral and manual), the level of drawing ability, measures of hand strength and speed, speech perception, and so on, were administered. Other tests idiosyncratic to a specific question will be described in the appropriate chapter. Still others which were administered but are not pertinent to the questions asked in this monograph will not be described at all.

Intelligence tests

Until mid-1984, the Wechsler Adult Intelligence Scale (WAIS; Wechsler, 1955) was administered to most nonaphasic patients, but to conserve time, the Information and Picture Arrangement subtests were omitted. In the case of patients with a hemiparesis affecting the preferred hand, Digit Symbol was also omitted. Thus Full Scale IQs were calculated from the prorated scores.

Since 1984, the WAIS-Revised (WAIS-R; Wechsler, 1981) has been administered but only four subtests have been used. The Block Design and Object Assembly subtests have been administered to all patients after the first year or two of the investigation. Vocabulary and Digit Span of the Verbal Scale were also administered, but only to nonaphasic patients. Wechsler's population mean raw scores for the 1955 and 1981 versions of the two Performance tasks are almost identical (Block Design, 31–34 for both versions of the WAIS; Object Assembly, 31–33 for the WAIS and 32–33 for the WAIS-R). Consequently, our data for these two versions of the subtests were combined for most purposes. Raw scores will be presented for these, because the scaled scores have a limited range. Where age is an important factor, this was either tested statistically, or the data presented for different age groups.

Aphasia tests

Two tests were used to classify patients as aphasic or not, and to measure degree of aphasic disturbance. In the first year or two of the study, a patient might not have received either of these tests, yet be classified as aphasic if there was a gross speech disturbance apparent in conversation.

1. *Aphasia screening test.* This was based on Schuell's *Minnesota Test for Differential Diagnosis of Aphasia* (1974). (See Kimura, 1986, for details.) There were two components. The Receptive scale consisted of recognizing common words (Schuell A-1), identifying items named serially (Schuell A-4), and understanding sentences to which only a Yes or No answer need be given. Maximum score was 43. The Expressive scale comprised counting to 20 (Schuell C-5), naming the days of the week (Schuell C-6), and naming pictures (Schuell C-13). Maximum score was 47.

The maximum score for the two scales combined was thus 90. Patients achieving scores of 86 or less—that is, making more than three errors—were classified as aphasic.

2. *Modified Token test.* This was an abbreviated version of a test devised by deRenzi and Vignolo (1962). (See Kimura, 1986, for details.) Test materials were colored plastic chips of various shapes, and patients were given a series of instructions which required pointing to, or placement of, these chips. Instructions gradually increased in difficulty as the test progressed. This is a very demanding test of speech comprehension in that it has little redundancy. Maximum score is 84, and a score of 75 or less classified a patient as aphasic.

A patient was classified as aphasic if the score was below the cutoff on *either* of the above tests.

Fluency/nonfluency. Immediately after the Expressive scale outlined above, the patient was asked to describe a complex picture (Schuell C-12), and a measure of speech fluency was derived from the recorded utterances (Goodglass, Quadfasel, & Timberlake, 1964). (See Kimura, 1986, for details.) This test was administered to all aphasics in order to classify the aphasia as fluent or nonfluent.

Apraxia tests

These were test in which postures or movements demonstrated live by the examiner had to be imitated by the patient. Tests in which movements were elicited by verbal command were discontinued after the first few years, since they had certain disadvantages (see Chapter 6 for details).

Oral movements. There were two levels of imitation: (1) Single oral movements, in which the patient reproduced, one at a time, a series of simple individual movements such as lateralizing the tongue, opening the mouth, and so on; maximum score was 17. (2) Multiple oral movements, in which each trial consisted of three oral movements and the patient was required to reproduce all three; several such trials were given; maximum score was 9. (See Kimura, 1986, for details.)

Manual movements. Whenever possible, both hands were tested. Again, there were two levels of movement required: (1) Single hand postures, in which static hand postures were demonstrated for imitation, such as closed fist, open hand, and so on; maximum score was 10. (2) Copying movements, in which each trial consisted of a series of movements involving one hand and arm, reproduction of which was scored in detail for hand posture, orientation with respect to the body, accuracy of movement, and so forth; maximum score was 24; a patient was designated as manually *apraxic* if the score was less than 13. (See Kimura, 1986, for details.)

In order to judge whether the limb contralateral to the lesion had adequate strength and motility to enable the copying of manual movements, two additional measures were taken of each hand: (1) hand strength as measured with a dynamometers and (2) finger tapping speed. (See Kimura, 1986, for details.)

A third test of manual apraxia was administered for a period of time, involving the acquisition of a manual skill on a box devised for this purpose (Kimura, 1977). A series of movements directed to various features of the box was demonstrated and then had to be learned by the patient, to a specified criterion (see Chapter 6 for details).

Hand preference

The patient was asked to demonstrate how to do eight different unimanual tasks (Kimura, 1986), including writing. To be classified as right-handed, a patient must write and do six of the seven remaining tasks with the right hand. All others were classed as adextral. Patients with hemiparesis were simply asked about their prior hand use on the same tasks, and for aphasic patients a close family member was questioned.

Speech reproduction

Simple reproduction of orally presented speech sounds was required in two levels: (1) *Single speech sounds*—one syllable was presented at a time and the patient simply repeated back the sound—for example, "s," "p." Included were vowels, fricatives, sibilants, liquids, and stop consonants. Each sound was scored as wrong or right, with a maximum score of 20. (2) Meaningful *multisyllabic phrases* were presented for the patient to repeat back—as, for example, "much food," "saves time." Each phrase was scored for number of individual phonemes correct, maximum score being 54.

In addition to these simple repetition tasks, a task was given in which the subject was to repeat syllables over and over as quickly as possible, called *speeded repetition.* In the first phase of the task, a single syllable was to be repeated over and over ("ba," and in a separate trial "ga"). The score was the mean number of correct syllables in 5 sec. In the second phase, the subject had to repeat the three-syllable utterance, "ba-da-ga," as quickly as possible. The score again was the number of individual syllables repeated in 5 sec, but in correct sequence.

Speech perception

Two tasks were presented, both employing the six stop consonants—"ba," "da," "ga," "pa," "ta," "ka." Some of the syllables were natural speech, others were computer-generated[1] and were deliberately constructed to have a voice-onset time which was between 20 and 30 msec off the peak natural onset time. (1) *Syllable identification*—each of the six syllables was played four times, in random order, and the patient responded by pointing to the corresponding syllable on a printed card containing all six. Maximum score was 24. (2) *Syllable discrimination*—two successive syllables had to be discriminated as same or different, a d' measure being used to derive a discrimination score.

Summary

This chapter introduces the idea that human communication has been shaped by the characteristics of the motor programming systems controlling the relevant musculature. That a complex manual system of communication may have preceded a complex vocal system is suggested by several lines of evidence from comparative and evolutionary studies.

Some of the limitations of previous research on the neural basis of human communication are outlined. In particular, selected case studies tend to give us incomplete information because they are not balanced by reference to other (negative) cases with similar nervous system pathology. Moreover, functional dissociations derived from single-case studies selected by symptomatology tend to be exaggerated. The neurological subjects of this book were selected solely on the basis of unilateral cerebral pathology, without reference to symptoms. They represent as unbiased a series of patients as is possible with consenting human subjects.

Notes

1. This tape was constructed by Jonathan Lomas with the assistance of Dr. Donald Shankweiler at the Haskins Laboratories, New Haven, Connecticut in 1978.

2. Asymmetry

The left and right cerebral hemispheres in people mediate quite different behavioral functions, and this phenomenon is referred to as *functional* brain asymmetry. Although the asymmetry of the two cerebral hemispheres relates to many functions besides communication, it was originally established as a fact within the context of speech disorders after left-hemisphere pathology. For many people, the raison d'être of cerebral asymmetry is the organization of language functions in one hemisphere, usually the left. The functions of the right hemisphere have been labeled "nonverbal" as a convenient contrast. Brain asymmetry is often viewed as associated with the presence of uniquely human or "higher-level" cognitive functions. That this is not the case is suggested by several lines of evidence: the pervasiveness of systematic asymmetry outside the nervous system; the fact of anatomical and functional brain asymmetry in nonhuman animals; the predisposition of the left hemisphere in humans to support all manner of speech-related functions, even such fundamental functions as voice volume and respiratory control; the evidence that complementary asymmetry is at least as reliable in very basic perceptual and motor processes as in so-called higher level processes; and so on.

Neural asymmetry in birds

In reviewing the evidence for functional asymmetry of the nervous system in nonhuman animals, we find that some of the strongest and most consistent asymmetries have been demonstrated in birds. Nottebohm (1981) has shown that a portion of the peripheral nervous system in canaries and chaffinches is very asymmetrically organized for singing. Thus the left hypoglossal nerve is paramount for the control of singing, which normally occurs only in males. If the left hypoglossal is cut, there is either no sound produced at all, or merely isolated clicks and distorted sounds, whereas sectioning of the right hypoglossal has no audible effect. The right hypoglossal can, however, mediate song if the left is cut in the first two weeks after hatching.

The evidence for functional *brain* asymmetry in birds is somewhat less striking than the hypoglossal asymmetry. When retrograde degeneration from sectioning the hypoglossal is traced back into the brain, there are several nuclei which are affected. The region most involved in song control is HVc (referring to "higher vocal center," according to

Nottebohm, 1987). Lesions of the left HVc result in significantly altered song, either in a complete loss, or with only a small segment remaining; while lesions of the right HVc result in no or minor audible changes. Spectrographic analyses, however, show less significant asymmetries after HVc lesions than after hypoglossal sectioning. Moreover, birds with HVc lesions recover significantly more song after several months than do birds with left hypoglossal section.

Why this striking asymmetry should be present in songbirds is not clear. It apparently is not related to extent of song learning, since noise-reared and deafened birds show the same pattern of dominance. Moreover, there is no such asymmetry in parrots, who acquire a much more extensive repertoire, which is more experientially based. Yet parrots are claimed to show a systematic foot preference for perching as opposed to food grasping (Harris, 1989).

Functional asymmetry in birds is by no means limited to song production. Andrew (1983) has shown that novelty, attack and fear responses are more likely to occur in the domestic chick when left-eye systems are being employed. Since the visual pathways in birds are almost entirely crossed, this means that the right brain hemisphere is more engaged in such situations than is the left. In contrast, fine discriminations, as between different kinds of potential food grains, is performed better by right-eye systems, engaging the left hemisphere. Rogers (1989) has demonstrated that such asymmetry can be altered by shifting the chick embryo before hatching, so that light comes atypically into the other eye. It is unclear whether the light is having an effect on peripheral visual systems primarily, or affecting basic hypothalamic systems with secondary effects on vision. Indeed, one might raise the question with all reports of bird asymmetry, whether the central nervous system lateralization is perhaps secondary to peripheral asymmetry.

Asymmetry in nonhuman mammals

In mammals, research has concentrated on primates, but there is evidence that cats show significantly functional, as well as anatomical, asymmetry, if one defines the hemispheres vis-à-vis the preferred paw rather than as left or right. Webster (1972) demonstrated that the learning of a series of visual discriminations in cats had in fact been more vested in one hemisphere than the other. He had ingeniously defined the hemispheres, however, as ipsilateral or contralateral to the preferred paw. After the cats had learned the discriminations in the normal way, either with an apparatus where they had to reach with the paw, or with one where a whole-body movement had to be made, he sectioned the corpus callosum and the optic chiasm. This produced a preparation in which there were only ipsilateral eye–brain connections.

Consequently, testing of the left eye was essentially equivalent to testing the left hemisphere. He found, during postoperative retraining on these tasks, that it was the hemisphere ipsilateral to the preferred paw which was superior. That is, if the cat had been right-pawed, the right hemisphere was superior. The data suggest complementary specialization between hemispheres in the cat, in that one hemisphere controls limb movements, while the other is important for processing external visual input. This is roughly analogous to functional asymmetry in humans in that the right hemisphere in most right-handers is superior for certain visuospatial functions.

A possibly related finding, also in cats, was reported by Robinson and Voneida (1973). In two normal cats in which the paw preference was not reported, there appeared to be right-hemisphere preference for doing visual discrimination tasks, as evidenced by superior performance when using the left eye (in cats the crossed pathways from eye to brain predominate). After the callosum was sectioned, this left-eye superiority was exaggerated, presumably due to reduced interference from the left hemisphere. However, when the chiasm was subsequently sectioned, there was a right-eye superiority, since the right eye now had exclusive access to the right hemisphere. Although we do not have paw preference information in the Robinson study, and the authors did not discuss this finding in terms of hemispheric preference for these tasks, the data are compatible with Webster's.

Gazzaniga (1963) reported essentially similar effects in three monkeys, all of whom happened to be right-handed. Visual discrimination habits learned in the normal state were found, after sectioning of the callosum, anterior commissure, and chiasm, to be organized primarily in the right hemisphere. All three of these studies suggest that even when a habit is learned with an intact normal brain, it is laid down in, or critically dependent on, one hemisphere more than another.

Recent systematic studies on a larger sample of Rhesus monkeys have suggested that opposing hemispheric asymmetries may exist for different types of visual stimuli (Hamilton & Vermeire, 1988*a*, 1988*b*). These investigators found, in monkeys whose brains were split before training, that perception of line orientation depended selectively on the left hemisphere, whereas facial discrimination depended on the right hemisphere. These effects were independent of handedness. This study is the only one to date showing convincing complementary specialization of function in the two hemispheres in nonhuman primates. The findings provide strong support for other evidence that brain asymmetry is not tied to the presence of human-type language.

Morphological anatomical asymmetries analogous to those found in humans have also been demonstrated in nonhuman primates. (See deLacoste, Horvath, & Woodward, 1988, for a more complete summary.)

Since it is often difficult in humans to evaluate the significance of morphological asymmetries until we have some demonstration of their behavioral relevance, their pertinence in nonhumans is even more problematic. The Sylvian fissure is known to extend further back in the left hemisphere than the right before rising dorsally in most people (Rubens, Mahowald, & Hutton, 1976), paralleling a larger area of planum temporale on the left (Geschwind & Levitsky, 1968). The latter is presumed to relate to the importance of this region for speech processing. The finding that the temporal-plane asymmetry is present and equivalent to the adult in infant and fetal brains (Wada, Clarke, & Hamm, 1975) indicates that it precedes any exposure to speech perception or production.

A Sylvian-fissure asymmetry similar to that described by Rubens and coworkers has been described in chimpanzees, though it is somewhat less marked than in humans (Yeni-Komshian & Benson, 1976). In Rhesus monkeys there was no significant difference between the hemispheres on this measure. Other systematic asymmetries, though not necessarily analogous to human patterns, have been reported in gorillas (Groves & Humphrey, 1973), Old World monkeys (Falk, 1978), baboons (Cain & Wada, 1979), and cats (Webster, 1981). A more recent study reports systematic intraspecies asymmetry in various lemur species (deLacoste, Horvath, & Woodward, 1988). This asymmetry varies in degree, and with direction along the anterior–posterior dimension, but is most common in the occipital cortex.

No adequate studies exist on possible functional asymmetry in chimpanzee or gorilla, largely because these animals are highly valued by human experimenters, and extremely expensive to obtain and maintain, making brain surgery as a method of investigation unpalatable. Only if some of the well-studied chimpanzees ultimately have unilateral strokes are we likely to gain some knowledge of chimpanzee brain function in this respect!

The nature of human brain asymmetry

There is an immense literature on human functional brain asymmetry. The earliest evidence for such asymmetry was the report by Dax and Broca in the 1860s of speech disorders after left-hemisphere pathology. This was not followed by comparable evidence of right-hemisphere specialization until the 1940s (e.g., Paterson & Zangwill, 1944). About 100 years after Dax and Broca, techniques were developed that permitted the detection of asymmetry in normal persons: first, the relating of differential ear superiorities in dichotic listening to hemispheric specialization for speech representation and melodic processing (Kimura, 1961, 1964); then the relating of differential visual-field superiorities for verbal and nonverbal material to hemispheric asymmetry (Kimura, 1966). Since the discovery of these perceptual techniques, a wealth of data has accumulated based on such normal asymmetries (see Bryden, 1982, for review).

While the first demonstration of a perceptual asymmetry unequivocally related to hemispheric asymmetry was the right-ear superiority for words (Kimura, 1961), it soon became apparent that such right-ear effects could be obtained for very simple consonant–vowel syllables that had no meaning, whereas there was no such superiority for steady-state vowels (Shankweiler & Studdert-Kennedy, 1967). This suggests that merely carrying a linguistic message, which vowels do as well as consonants, does not result in asymmetric processing.

Similarly, left visual-field superiorities, indicating preferential right-hemisphere processing, have been shown to be reliable for simple perceptual processes such as dot location, dot enumeration, and perception of line slant (Kimura & Durnford, 1974). They tend not to occur for perception of shapes, whether upright or inverted, or for complex patterned matrices. While some of the latter failures of perceptual asymmetry may be related to the different brain areas involved in processing complex shapes as compared to simple stimuli, the findings nevertheless do not support the idea that asymmetry occurs only in later more cognitive stages of processing (Moscovitch, 1979).

The phenomenon of hand preference is another pervasive example of asymmetry detectable in normal people. That over 90% of the population is right-handed was originally interpreted as stemming from the left hemisphere's "dominance" over the right. Later work demonstrated that the left hand was actually better than the right, in right-handers, in performing certain fine motor tasks (Kimura & Vanderwolf, 1970; Ingram, 1975). Again the division of labor does not easily fit the idea of a distinction between two higher-level cognitive functions. Chapter 9 in fact presents evidence that hand preference may be based on similar motor-programming mechanisms in dextrals and adextrals, though represented in opposite hemispheres.

Mechanisms of brain asymmetry

Although it has been assumed in the past that brain asymmetry is a feature especially of cortical systems, evidence is accumulating that systematic asymmetry is an almost universal feature of biological systems. Human fetal gonads (both ovaries and testes) are larger on the right than on the left; and in adult males, testes are also significantly larger on the right than the left, in both Orientals and Caucasians (Mittwoch, 1988). Mittwoch (1976; Mittwoch & Madadevaiah, 1980) also reports that, when there are anomalies in gonadal development, the left gonad is significantly more likely to become an ovary, and the right to become a testis. For example, this trend becomes manifest in some human hermaphrodites. In birds, only the left ovary is typically functional, the right remaining vestigial.

Gerendai (1987) reviews evidence for endocrine asymmetry in a number of species, and specifically describes studies showing gonadal asymmetry in endocrine function in rats. There appears also to be a strong ipsilateral gonad–hypothalamic axis in regulation of hormonal release (Mizunuma, DePalatis, & McCann, 1983; Gerendai, 1987), suggesting that the hypothalamus may also function asymmetrically. The evidence favoring an ipsilateral influence implies a neural connection, since the systemic blood supply would foster more generalized effects.

Direct evidence that the hypothalamus functions asymmetrically in behavior comes from a study by Nordeen and Yahr (1982). Treatment with androgens, male sex hormones, pre- or perinatally in rodents is known to result in masculinization of the brain (Goy & McEwen, 1980). Some of this effect depends on the fact that androgens may be converted to estradiol, a female sex hormone, in the nervous system. Female infants are normally protected from such masculinization by the systemic presence of α-fetoprotein. In the Nordeen and Yahr study, estrogen was implanted directly into either the left or the right hypothalamus of newborn female rats, thus circumventing the systemic defense system. Treatment of the left hypothalamus resulted in "defeminization"—that is, reduced lordosis as an adult; whereas treatment of the right side resulted in increased "masculinization," thus increased mounting as an adult.

The previous studies suggest that certain aspects of male and female sexual behaviour are asymmetrically mediated in the hypothalamus. By implication, other hemispheric asymmetries may be a secondary consequence of such hypothalamic asymmetry, or both may reflect a general tendency, evident also in somatic asymmetry, for the two sides to be different. The greater thickness of the right cortex in male rodents (Diamond, Dowling, & Johnson, 1981) may be part of this picture.

Asymmetries analogous to those in rodents have recently been reported in human fetal brains. That is, males tend to have a more voluminous right cortex, while females show no difference between hemispheres, or have a tendency for the left cortex to be slightly greater in area (deLacoste, Horvarth, & Woodward, 1991). These findings have generally been interpreted to be specific to the nervous system, suggesting that testosterone, an important male sex hormone, alters the direction of brain asymmetry (Geschwind & Galaburda, 1984). Stewart and Kolb's (1988) data in rodents suggest that the presence of androgens can have a suppressive effect on left-hemisphere growth.

Somatic asymmetry in humans

There are, however, reasons for thinking that many aspects of lateral asymmetry may originate in cytoplasmic activity, and that they may antedate the presence of sex-determining hormones. Initial growth in the embryo may in fact first favor the left side, and later the right (Corballis & Beale, 1976). Indeed, differences in the rate of embryonic growth in the right-favoring period have been suggested as a mechanism for sexual differentiation, with more rapid growth favoring testicular development (Mittwoch, 1985, 1988). Obviously, testosterone would not be produced until after testicular differentiation, thus it could not be the basis for the gonadal asymmetry, though it could conceivably enhance other aspects of somatic and brain asymmetry in later stages.

Levy and Levy (1978) proposed that testosterone affected not only brain but also body asymmetry. They reported that direction of asymmetry in foot size was different in human males and females, favoring the left in females and the right in males. The finding of a sex difference in foot asymmetry has unfortunately failed to be replicated by others, including ourselves. It nevertheless remains an intriguing possibility that there might be individual differences in body asymmetry, related to factors such as sex and hand preference. Accordingly, as part of a larger study, we asked normal young undergraduates to do a self-inspection of asymmetries in testicular or breast size (ovaries are clearly not available for self-inspection!). The results were entirely consonant with Levy's report on foot size. More males reported being larger on the right, in agreement with reports in the literature (Mittwoch, 1988), and more females reported being larger on the left (Table 2.1). While it is true that comparing breast and testis sizes is problematic, both are known to be under the influence of sex hormones.

It is of course tempting to speculate that brain asymmetries will parallel such body asymmetries, but we have at present no direct information on this question. However, even if adult human males have a significantly thicker right cortex, and so far we have information only in fetal human brains, implications for *functional* brain asymmetry are

Table 2.1 Results of self-inspection of testicular or breast asymmetry in normal young adults

Sex	Left larger	Same	Right larger
Males (108)	25	36	47
Females (112)	42	51	19

not straightforward. We will discuss individual differences in brain organization, including the effects of sex and hand preference, in Chapters 9 and 10. It will then become clear that we do not find strong evidence for sex differences in functional brain asymmetry. Thus it may be that somatic, and even cortical-thickness asymmetries, are indices only of more rapid growth in some periods of embryonic development than others, rather than direct indices of functional brain organization.

We have thus outlined some evidence that systematic asymmetry is not specific to the nervous system; nor within the nervous system, exclusive to human beings. It is also evident that the specialized functions of the two hemispheres cannot be simply reduced to language and nonlanguage systems. In Chapter 3 we will see that the left hemisphere, known to be critical for speech, mediates a variety of low-level elementary speech functions, and that such asymmetry is not limited to cerebral cortex.

Summary

Lateralization of function in the brain is neither unique to humans nor specifically tied to the presence of complex language or other "higher level" functions. In fact, asymmetry is a feature of many biological systems, and is most marked in birds. It is suggested that neural lateralization may be secondary to other, possibly gonadal, asymmetries. The latter may also relate to possible sex differences in somatic and brain asymmetry.

3. Noncortical systems in speaking

Traditional views of the critical importance to speech of Wernicke's and Broca's cortical areas tend to downplay the important contributions of other brain regions. If we ask instead, what neuroanatomical systems are involved in speech in the sense that (1) damage to them produces impairment in speaking or (2) electrical stimulation influences or produces speech output, then we must conclude that wide areas of the brain are involved in the production of speech. Within the left cerebral cortex, the *entire peri-Sylvian region is involved in the production of speech* if we keep in mind that errors of speaking are produced in Wernicke's aphasia, as well as in Broca's aphasia. Moreover, the left-hemisphere's preeminence for speech control is not limited to the cortex, but appears in noncortical speech systems such as the thalamus, basal ganglia, and cerebellum. In addition, this hemispheric asymmetry is evident in basic speech functions, such as the control of voice volume and breathing.

Lower motor systems in speaking

Peripheral innervation of the speech musculature

Since speech involves activity of the larynx, palate, tongue, lips and jaw, as well as of the thorax, it is obvious that damage to the cranial nerves innervating these structures will have an effect on speech. The cranial nerves chiefly involved in speech are motor fibres of the trigeminal (V), facial (VII), vagus (X), accessory (XI), and hypoglossal (XII) nerves (Hollien, 1975) (Fig. 3.1).

Peripheral damage to any of these nerves is nearly always unilateral, and movements in speaking can therefore be compensated by the intact nerves on the other side. Thus unilateral damage to the facial nerve causes paresis of the muscles on one side of the face, but while speech is certainly changed in character, intelligibility remains good. Unilateral damage to the vagus nerve, which innervates the larynx and pharynx, may cause a change in voice quality, since one vocal cord does not adduct properly. However, the other vocal chord tends to compensate for this by adducting across the midline, and the only sign in speech may be a slight weakness in speaking or a tendency to fatigue. Damage to the hypoglossal nerve on one side may cause the tongue to deviate, but again, intelligibility remains high. More commonly, several cranial

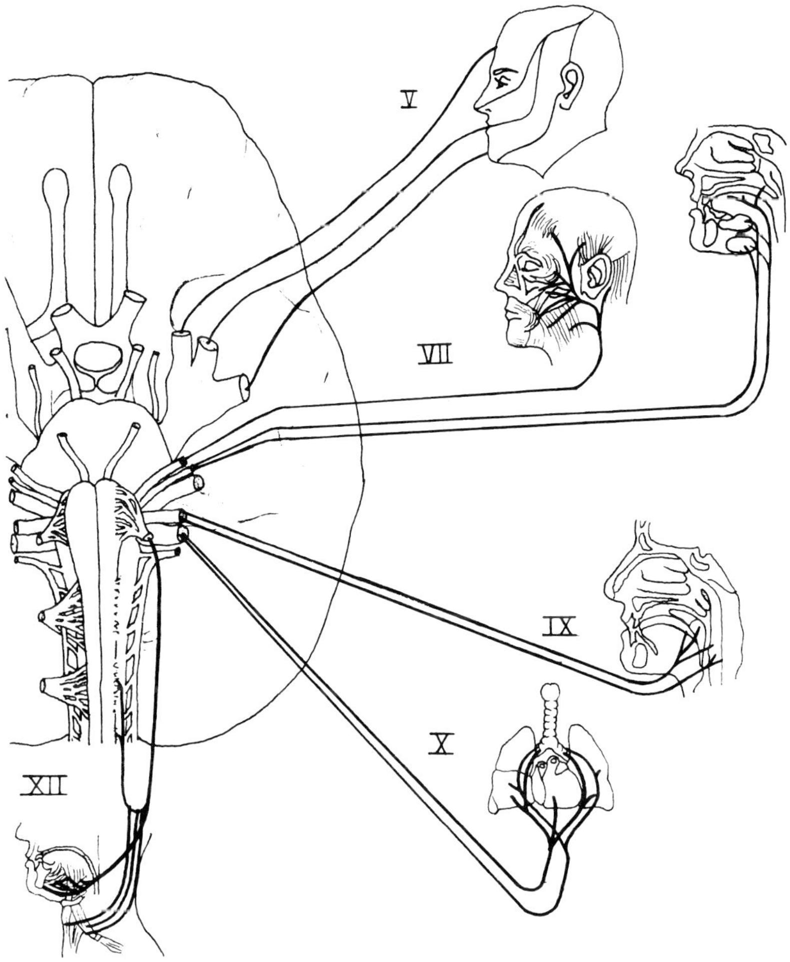

Fig. 3.1 Cranial nerves involved in speaking. V (trigeminal)—sensory to face; VII (facial)—motor innervation of facial muscles, sensory to soft palate; IX (glossopharyngeal)—sensory and motor to tongue and pharynx; X (vagus)—bronchial tubes, larynx and pharynx; XII (hypoglossal)—muscles of tongue.

nerves which travel together may be affected on one side—for example, IX, X, and XI—but even here compensation by the contralateral musculature is sufficient to attain intelligible speech.

Bilateral damage to the cranial nerves involved in speech most commonly occurs in lesions affecting more than one nerve. This makes it difficult to define the relative role of individual cranial nerve nuclei in speech control. It is nevertheless clear that complete bilateral paralysis of the larynx still permits intelligible whispering, sometimes by expulsion of air through the folds of the pharynx. In contrast, bilateral paralysis of the tongue may severely affect articulation, in that the lingual consonants ("t," "d," "td") and anteriorly placed vowels (such as the vowel in "beet") are affected. A general conclusion from the data on speech pathology is that the laryngeal contribution to speaking, though unequivocally important for communicating over a distance, is less critical for intelligibility than the lingual and labial contribution.

Bulbar palsy

Where progressive motor neuron disease is predominantly of muscles innervated from the medulla, the term "bulbar palsy" is usually applied. The effects on speech are presumed to be due to lesions of the respective cranial nerve nuclei in the medulla. The kind of speech disorder seen in bulbar palsy is usually described as "flaccid dysarthria." It is characterized by hypernasality (due to involvement of the palate), imprecise consonants (lip and tongue involvement), breathy voice (poor laryngeal control), and monopitch (see Darley, Aronson, & Brown, 1975). Ultimately, there is wasting of the muscles innervated by the affected neurons.

Since the lesions are almost never unilateral, although the symptoms may be asymmetric, and since the extent of the pathology at any one point in the progression of symptoms is generally unknown, it is not possible to make any statement about asymmetry of vocal control at the medullary level. There may or may not be such asymmetry.

Pseudobulbar palsy

Pseudobulbar palsy is so-called because the paresis is imitative of bulbar palsy, but the absence of muscular wasting, and the presence of spasticity, indicates that the lesion is antecedent to the final common path, i.e., supranuclear. The effects on speech are thus a consequence of weakness of the musculature, combined with increased spasticity or tone. Speech in pseudobular palsy will again show imprecise consonants and monopitch, but in addition there is a crying or strained quality to the voice (see Darley, Aronson, & Brown, 1975), reflecting the spastic component. The location of pathology may be anywhere between cortex and medulla. Pseudobulbar speech or spastic dysarthria is frequently associated with sudden spasms of laughing or crying, suggesting that in such cases a general system responsible for oral-facial control is affected. Brodal (1981) interprets such outbursts as a loss of inhibition from cortex to these centers, which is also the mechanism proposed for the spasticity. Again we have no conclusive information on whether there is asymmetry of speech control at these levels.

Thalamus and basal ganglia systems

Most of our information concerning the role of subcortical systems subserving speech has come from patients in whom stereotaxic lesions of thalamus or basal ganglia were carried out in an attempt to alleviate movement disorders. In the course of exploring the brain for an effective lesion, the neurosurgeon stimulates various regions through an electrode which will ultimately be the vehicle for making the lesion. The most common sites for therapeutic lesions of this type have been the globus pallidus, and the nucleus ventralis lateralis of the thalamus. Systematic studies of speech during stimulation have been uncommon, however, and even the effects of lesions on speech have generally come from retrospective studies. When we consider that many patients with movement disorders, particularly Parkinsonism, already have speech disorders before surgery, the problems in evaluating the effects of lesions on speech are evident. On the other hand, perhaps because of the very nature of the pretreatment speech difficulties present in this clinical population, investigators have taken a broader look at speech control than is often the case in cortical damage, and have included such measures as voice volume, breathing control, and articulation, as well as more usual tasks such as naming. We will first consider the evidence from stimulation studies, then the effects of lesions.

Stimulation studies

Figure 3.2 depicts the chief thalamo-cortical projections pertinent to the stimulation studies. Nucleus ventralis lateralis (Vl) projects to primary motor cortex or precentral gyrus (Brodmann's area 4), while ventralis anterior (Va) projects to premotor cortex (areas 6 and 8). The

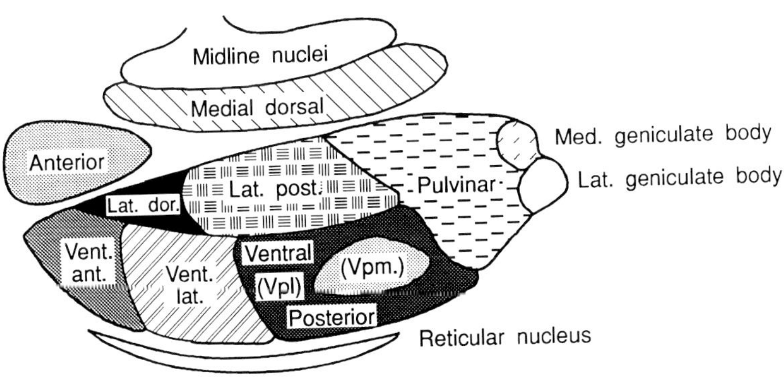

Fig. 3.2 Thalamo-cortical projection systems relevant to speech: ventralis anterior, ventralis lateralis, pulvinar.

other major thalamic nucleus we will discuss is the pulvinar, which projects to temporo-parietal cortex.

The effects of stimulation can be roughly divided into three main classes—production or acceleration of speech, arrest or slowing of speech, and actual errors in speech.

Production and acceleration

Acceleration of counting during stimulation has been reported by Guiot, Hertzog, Rondot, and Molina (1961), especially when the stimulating electrode is in Vl of the thalamus. Such acceleration is usually accompanied by a decrease in voice volume, with the last few numbers "lost in inarticulate stammering." Acceleration may be produced by stimulation at the same point, in the same patient (though on different occasions), which produces arrest of counting. Since the acceleration often ends in a stifled voice and complete stoppage of speech, it appears that the speech musculature is driven faster but with less exhalation force than usual. Guiot and coworkers claim that these effects can occur with or without tetanizing contractions of the face. They do not compare the incidence of these effects from left- and right-sided stimulations.

The only comparable effect in other stimulation studies has been the report of acceleration in backward counting during stimulation of Vl, and possibly decreased latency in naming (Ojemann, 1976).

Production of speech was reported by Schaltenbrand (1965), during stimulation of what was probably nucleus ventralis anterior (German terminology, ventralis oralis anterior; see Crosby, Humphrey, & Laurer, 1962, p. 286). Coherent speech, which bore no relation to the context, was forced by the stimulation, and even if the patient was asked not to talk, he still did so. This is in sharp contrast to the effect of cortical stimulation, which has *never* been reported to produce an intelligible speech sound. The number of patients studied by Schaltenbrand was small, but there is the suggestion that speech is more often produced by left thalamic stimulation than by right (50% versus 14%). The only comparable effect in other studies is the report of rare extraneous verbalizations during left Vl stimulation (Ojemann, 1976) (Table 3.1).

Arrest and slowing

In contrast to cortical stimulation, simple arrest or cessation has been infrequently reported from thalamic stimulation. Guiot and coworkers (1961) have produced arrest from the same points as they produced acceleration (see above), suggesting some overdriving of the system.

Ojemann (1976) and his coworkers have reported the effects of stimulation within a paradigm in which the patient is shown a picture of a familiar object, and must say "This is a ———" and the name of the object. Simple arrest is defined in this context as an inability to

Table 3.1 Effects of stimulating thalamus and basal ganglia

Change in speech	Site	Occurrence		Source
		Left	Right	
Arrest	Caudate nucleus	6/?	2/?	Van Buren (1963)
Slowing	Ventralis lateralis	60% increase	2% increase	Mateer (1978)
Acceleration while counting	Ventralis lateralis	Sides not compared		Guiot and coworkers (1961)
Production of coherent speech	Ventralis anterior	50%	14%	Schaltenbrand (1965)
Misnaming	Ventralis lateralis	50%	7%	Ojemann (1976)
Anomia	Pulvinar	77%	0%	Ojemann (1976)

produce the phrase during stimulation. Few such cessations of speech occur, but this may in part be due to the fact that the phrase "This is a" is produced dozens of times in the course of the study, and therefore might be less subject to interference than more spontaneous speech, even counting. The few sites which do show arrest do not suggest asymmetry between left and right sides.

A follow-up study by Mateer (1978) on some of Ojemann's data is of interest, however. She analyzed tapes of patients being stimulated in the Vl nucleus of the thalamus during the paradigm described above. Restricting herself to trials where the correct name was produced by the patient, she found that stimulation nevertheless prolonged the duration of the utterance during left, but not right thalamic stimulation. Some of the increase in time was apparently reflected in audible "slurring and articulatory distortion." This effect is unequivocal, in that it was evaluated statistically over a number of patients, but it is difficult to reconcile with Ojemann's claim that left thalamic stimulation decreases naming latency.

The clearest report of arrest of speech from subcortical stimulation comes from stimulation of the caudate nucleus by Van Buren (1963). It is not clear how patients were chosen for report, but presumably because they showed changes in speech. The arrest was evident as simple cessation of counting. Of the eight cases described, six were left-sided, two right. In both the right-sided cases, there was head and eye turning to the left during arrest, whereas in only one of the six left-sided cases was there associated head and eye turning. On at least one occasion, a patient who could not count spontaneously during stimulation, could repeat words. Since repetition of speech has not been systematically tested in other brain stimulation studies, we have no way of knowing how it compares with spontaneous speech in susceptibility to disruption by brain stimulation. It would be expected, from the aphasia literature, that it would generally be less affected than spontaneous speech.

Errors in speaking

Most of the work, and all of the systematic work, on errors in speaking during thalamic stimulation has been done by Ojemann and his coworkers. The typical procedure has been described above: the presentation of a picture, with the requirement that the patient say the phrase "This is a ———" and the name. Anomic errors are defined as those in which the carrying phrase is repeated correctly, but the patient either gives no name or a wrong name, or occasionally, repeats the first syllable of the correct name. This is thus roughly comparable to the category "inability to name with retained ability to speak," used by Penfield and Roberts (1959).

With stimulation of the Vl nucleus on the left, anomic errors occurred approximately half the time, but on the right occurred infrequently (Ojemann, 1976). Later reports by Ojemann suggested even greater asymmetry when stimulating the pulvinar: 15 of 18 left-sided electrodes yielded anomic responses, while none of the 16 right-sided electrodes did so (Ojemann, 1977). The type of naming error also differentiates these two sites. Thus, the more anterior region of Vl has produced misnamings which are perseverations on the first syllable of the target word; whereas the more posterior part of Vl, adjacent to the pulvinar, and the pulvinar itself, give rise to whole-word errors and omissions (Ojemann, 1983). It would be interesting to compare the effects of anterior and posterior cortical stimulation in this respect, but unfortunately, Penfield and Roberts' data are not broken down in a way which yields word and syllable repetitions separately.

Ojemann and Van Buren (1967) had earlier found that sites in the left Vl and pulvinar which yielded speech disorders, also had lower thresholds for changes in respiration than corresponding sites on the right. They speculated that this was related to some general integrative function of the left thalamus in the control of speaking. In any case, it is clear that stimulation of the left thalamus yields a variety of changes in speech which range from the so-called "higher order" functions such as naming, to very basic functions such as speed of speaking, articulatory control, and respiration. Thus even the most elementary kinds of vocal control appear to be asymmetrically organized in the brain. Data from thalamic lesions, reviewed below, confirm and extend these conclusions.

Lesion studies

Studies on the effects of subcortical lesions on speech involve essentially the same population as those in whom the effects of stimulation are studied, i.e., primarily patients with movement disorders undergoing stereotaxic surgery. Spontaneously occurring thalamic lesions, which can be identified during the life of the patient, do sometimes occur and can add to our knowledge of the effects of damage.

The effects on speech which have been described after thalamic lesions include diminution in voice volume, reduction in fluency, articulatory difficulty or dysarthria, and dysphasia, although the latter is not often described in detail.

Diminution in voice volume and fluency

Hermann, Turner, Gillingham, and Gaze (1966) report on the effects of subcortical lesions in a sizable number of patients. After left-sided operations, voice volume, measured by a sound intensity meter, was diminished in 67% of cases. After right-sided operations, only 36%

deteriorated in voice volume. Lesions were in the thalamus, the posterior limb of the internal capsule, or globus pallidus. A study by Bell (1968) on ventralis lateralis lesions showed a very similar picture: 45% of left-sided lesions resulted in reduced voice volume, while only 14% of right-sided lesions did so. When one considers that preexisting speech problems in these cases might mask the effects of subsequent surgery, these differences become more noteworthy.

A possibly related deficit seen after left thalamotomy is a reduction in speeded word fluency. Almgren, Andersson, and Kullberg (1969) reported that left-sided lesions resulted in a reduced number of correctly named colors within a specified time, under both a simple and complex condition. The left-sided cases differed in these respects from right-sided lesions. This impairment was still seen several months later, and was thus not due to dysfunction of neighboring edematous tissue (Almgren, Andersson & Kullberg, 1972). Riklan, Levita, Zimmermann, and Cooper (1969) found essentially the same effect of left Vl lesions on a task requiring the patient to say as many words as possible within a specified time period, beginning with a particular letter. Laitinen and Vilkki (1977) also reported deficits after left thalamic lesions on a word fluency task, and in the time taken to name simple colored shapes.

The interpretation generally put upon these data is that the deficits represent a fairly high-level intellectual impairment, but there is nothing in the facts themselves to suggest that there is anything more than a slowness in making a speaking response, particularly since the simplest color naming task in the Almgren study brought out the impairment. Unfortunately, no research has been done to relate changes in speaking latencies, speed of speaking, changes in voice volume, etc., to other verbal difficulties. (A mild verbal memory problem found in the Almgren study was no longer present several months later.) We cannot even tell, from these studies, whether the reduction in the amount or speed of speech is specific to speaking, or whether it extends to nonspeech activities as well. The generally lower incidence after right-sided lesions indirectly argues against such an explanation, but it does not rule it out (Table 3.2).

Articulatory difficulty

Often the impairments in this category are so meagerly described as to make it doubtful if they can be included in any category. Thus the term "dysarthria," unelaborated, may be used, or a statement made to the effect that a patient was "dysarthric" but not "dysphasic," when in fact the dividing line between the two is not always clear. Nevertheless, on the assumption that the term "dysarthria" usually includes slurring and distortion of speech sounds, the following statements may be made. Hermann and coworkers (1966) report that slurring, hesitation and

Table 3.2 Effects of lesions of thalamus and basal ganglia on volume and speed of speaking

Change in speech	Site	Occurrence		Source
		Left	Right	
Reduced voice volume	Thalamus, internal capsule globus pallidus	67%	36%	Hermann and coworkers (1966)
	Ventralis lateralis	45%	14%	Bell (1968)
	Thalamus	Single case, left		Fazio and coworkers (1973)
Fading voice volume	Thalamus	2 left-sided cases		Mohr and coworkers (1975)
Reduced speed of labeling	Ventralis lateralis	Left greater than right		Almgren and coworkers (1969)
Reduced word fluency	Ventralis lateralis	Left greater than right		Riklan and coworkers (1969)

Table 3.3 Effects of lesions of thalamus and basal ganglia on articulation and speech errors

Change in speech	Site	Occurrence		Source
		Left	Right	
Articulatory difficulty	Thalamus, internal capsule globus pallidus	54%	36%	Hermann and coworkers (1966)
Dysarthria	Ventralis lateralis	81%	32%	Bell (1968)
Dysphasic errors	Ventralis lateralis	Rare but greater on left		Ojemann (1976)
	Thalamus	Single case, left		Fazio and coworkers (1973)
	Thalamus	3/4 left-sided cases		Mohr and coworkers (1975)

occasional speeding up of speech are more often consequences of left-sided operations (54%) than of right-sided operations (36%). Bell (1968) reports a somewhat sharper separation between left and right surgery in that dysarthria occurred in 81% of left thalamotomies and in only 32% of right thalamotomies. In the Hermann study, it is not clear how comparable the lesions on the two sides were, and in the Bell study, no criteria for dysarthria are stated, but it appears, taking both together, that articulatory difficulties are more often a consequence of left-sided lesions.

Both Bell (1968) and Ojemann and Ward (1973) suggest that the dysarthria present after thalamotomies may be secondary to damage to the posterior limb of the internal capsule, which courses near the sites of the stereotaxic lesions. Hermann and coworkers also report that those left-sided lesions resulting in poorer articulation were often in the internal capsule, whereas this was not true of articulatory deterioration from right-sided lesions. The implication is that the dysarthric changes are due, not to thalamic damage per se, but to interruption of downgoing motor paths from the cortex. These opinions may represent an early bias about the relative contributions of thalamus and cortex, rather than an actual state of affairs. A slightly different bias probably underlies the claim by Riklan and coworkers (1969) that "speech" disorders, as compared with "language" disorders, are no more common after left-sided thalamic surgery than after right. Not enough data are presented to support the claim, and in view of the studies reported above, it appears most unlikely (Table 3.3).

Nonarticulatory errors in speech

A great deal of inference may go into the labeling of an error as "articulatory" versus "aphasic." For example, distortion of a syllable might be considered an articulatory error, but some such distortions could not be distinguished from the production of a different, inappropriate syllable. On the assumption that the term "dysphasia" generally refers to nonarticulatory errors primarily of the whole-word type, it appears that dysphasia is a relatively infrequent consequence of stereotaxic thalamic lesions. It occurs in 10–15% of cases, and nearly always transiently. When it does occur, it is claimed in all cases to be a consequence of left-sided lesions. Ojemann (1976) again provides the only systematic data, from his naming test. After thalamic Vl lesions, naming errors are more common and more severe when the lesion is on the left than when it is on the right.

It must be kept in mind that lesions made therapeutically for movement disorders have been primarily in ventralis lateralis and ventralis anterior of the thalamus, both of which project to the frontal lobe, the former to the motor, and the latter to the premotor cortex. It might therefore be expected that there is some similarity of thalamic function with the function of these cortical regions. This in fact seems to be true insofar as the relatively high incidence of articulatory versus nonarticulatory errors is concerned. (See the section on effects of stimulation of anterior cortex in Chapter 4.)

Stereotaxic lesions are not typically made in the thalamic nuclei which project to posterior cortex, e.g., in the pulvinar. Thalamic hemorrhages, on the other hand, necessarily involve much larger areas of the thalamus than does a stereotaxic lesion, and they may result in a variety of speech disorders. Fazio, Sacco, and Bugiani (1973) report on a case of hemorrhage, which postmortem pathology showed involved the whole thalamus on the left. The patient was sufficiently testable to establish that voice volume was low, but articulation and repetition of words were apparently normal. However, his spontaneous speech was "poor and full of syntactic errors, paraphasias and stereotypes." Mohr, Watters, and Duncan (1975) report on four cases in which pathology was determined by computed tomography scan or by postmortem examination of the brain. The speech deficits ranged from "mild dysarthria with aphasia" to "logorrheic paraphasia," with ability to repeat long complicated words. It is noteworthy that two patients had a combination of fading voice volume and jargonlike speech, but with apparently good articulation.

Although Mohr and coworkers felt that the dysphasic (as opposed to dysarthric) deficits depend on damage to the posterior nuclei, their data on pathology are not in strong support of this claim. The same may be said of the cases of Ciemins (1970), in that the one case in whom the speech disorder was sufficiently described had a hemorrhage involving the entire left thalamus. More recent studies also employing computed tomography scan determination of the locus of thalamic hemorrhage or infarct (Wallesch & coworkers, 1983; Cappa, Papagno, Vallar, & Vignolo, 1986), suggest that aphasia may be uncommon after restricted posterior thalamic damage involving the pulvinar. This is in apparent conflict with the high incidence of naming disorders upon stimulation of the left pulvinar (see Ojemann, 1977, above). Possibly it is the effect of pulvinar stimulation added to an already existing basal ganglia lesion in the movement disorder cases which accounts for this discrepancy. Although not enough is known at present about the details of speech disorders after thalamic lesions, there does not appear to be a simple correlation between the thalamic sites and the speech disorders found with lesions of their cortical projection areas. This would argue that the thalamic lesions are not having their effect solely by disruption of their connections to cortical speech areas.

Cerebellum

Disorders of speaking are quite common from cerebellar pathology, and they are similar to the disorders seen in other parts of the body, i.e., the rate and rhythm of the movements are disordered. Characteristically, the speech is monotonous, with unusual or unnatural separation of the syllables, resulting in slurred, jerky or explosive speech (Holmes, 1922). The term "ataxic dysarthria" has been used to label the speech disorders after cerebellar disease (Darley, Aronson, & Brown, 1975), which is described as showing "——irregular——breakdowns in articulatory precision."

A review of a large series of cases has uncovered a discrepancy between the incidence of speech disorders after left and right cerebellar lesions (Lechtenberg & Gilman, 1978). The incidence is significantly higher after lesions restricted to the left cerebellar hemisphere. The authors suggest that this asymmetry is related, not to left cerebral functioning for language, but rather to right cerebral specialization for analysis of prosody, or speech rhythm. (Since cerebro-cerebellar connections are apparently predominantly crossed, it is the right cerebral hemisphere which has the greater input to the left cerebellum.) The right cerebral hemisphere is claimed by some to contribute important noncontent parameters to speech analysis, such as emotional tone (Ley & Bryden, 1982; Ross, 1981; Shipley-Brown, Dingwall, Berlin, Yeni-Komshian, & Gordon-Salant, 1988), or even linguistic tone, such as declarative and interrogative characteristics (Shipley-Brown & coworkers, 1988).

However, in view of the overwhelming importance of the left cerebral hemisphere's contribution to normal prosody in speech *production* (Monrad-Krohn, 1947; Goodglass, Quadfasel, & Timberlake, 1964), Lechtenberg and Gilman's interpretation seems very unlikely. There is no evidence that the right cerebral hemisphere contributes significantly to speech production, even intonation. We also have no evidence that the cerebellum contributes to speech intonation–perception, though the disturbances in production of speech after cerebellar damage can be salient and severe. Whether the special contribution of the left cerebellum to speech is in some way related to the left cerebral hemisphere's specialization for speech control (perhaps via ipsilateral brainstem connections), or proceeds from some other intrinsic cerebellar asymmetry is at present an unsolved puzzle.

Summary

We have seen that functional brain asymmetry for the control of speech production is present in thalamus, basal ganglia, and cerebellum, not in cerebral cortex. Moreover, it appears to be present for the most elementary of speech-control features, including voice volume and rhythm. The noncortical contributions to speech control do not seem merely to mimic the function of the cortical regions with which they are connected, but show some distinctive characteristics. With this background, we will concentrate in Chapter 4 on speech functions dependent on the neocortex. Some of these functions overlap those of the systems we have reviewed in this chapter, whereas other features of cortical organization appear to have no simple parallel in subcortical systems.

4. Cortical systems in speaking

Investigation into the cortical systems involved in speaking has largely been a matter of describing speech disorders in individual cases of brain damage. Delineating the extent and locus of the underlying neural pathology has usually been attempted only with reference to positive instances of specified aphasic syndromes. The syndrome approach in aphasia has tended to maintain existing typologies, the components of the syndrome typically not being measured separately or objectively (e.g., production and comprehension in "Wernicke's" aphasia). Most studies have sought merely to reinforce a classification. The stultifying effect of this approach can be seen in the fact that essentially the same concepts are employed in aphasiology as existed at the turn of the century, with only one addition (fluency).

Of the plethora of aphasia classifications, the most durable are Broca's and Wernicke's, or their near synonyms, expressive and receptive aphasia, respectively. The premature acceptance of the simplistic model of language organization exemplified by this expressive/receptive dichotomy has probably been the single greatest impediment to the collection of meaningful data on speech mechanisms. The limitations of the initially productive ground-breaking formulations by Broca (translated in von Bonin, 1960) and Wernicke (1874) were pointed out early by Dejerine (1913) and von Monakow (1914); however these formulations nevertheless survived, and are still with us in modified form to this day.

The early work of Dax and Broca established that damage to parts of the left frontal lobe resulted in profound limitations in the production of speech; in contrast, comprehension of speech seemed relatively intact. Although the evidence for retention of comprehension in such cases was very patchy, it soon became axiomatic in the literature that left anterior lesions did not cause significant speech perception deficits. Wernicke's (1874) subsequent description of cases of posterior temporal-lobe damage, with clear comprehension difficulties but "preserved" speech production, seemed to confirm the anatomical separation of production and comprehension functions. This view persisted despite the many speech errors produced by "Wernicke's" aphasics. The latter, however, usually possessed an easy flow of speech, in contrast to the often labored articulation of patients with "Broca's" aphasia (Fig. 4.1).

Variations on these two major categories were soon proposed, e.g., "transcortical motor aphasia" (Lichtheim, 1885), in which repetition of

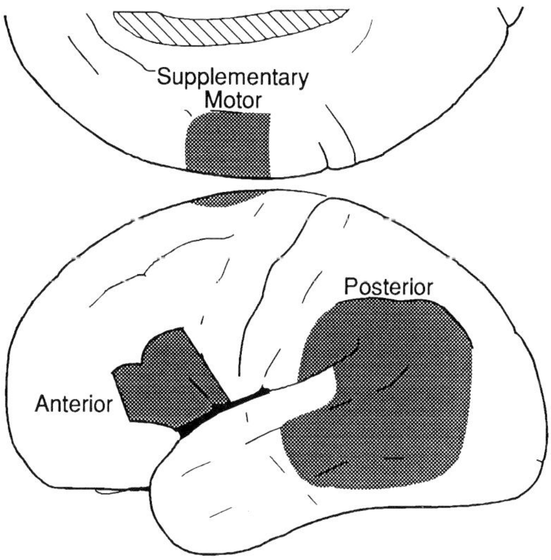

Fig. 4.1 Major speech areas on the cortical surface, determined from the effects of electrical stimulation. (After Penfield & Roberts, 1959.)

speech was apparently better than in classical Broca's aphasia. Many of these minor classifications, however, ignored the probability that not all production or comprehension tasks are of equivalent difficulty, and thus that not every apparent dissociation necessarily means a separable function. It is generally agreed that simple repetition of heard speech is easier than is the spontaneous production of speech, making it likely that categories like transcortical motor aphasia are simply milder forms of a Broca's aphasia (Freud, 1891). Classification of comprehension deficits also proliferated. "Transcortical sensory aphasia" (Lichtheim, 1885) was seen as separate from Wernicke's aphasia in that speech repetition was relatively unimpaired. Again, it is probable that difficulty level plays a role, in that repetition may recover earlier or more readily than other speech functions (Bastian & Lond, 1897; Brown, 1972).

Similarly, "conduction aphasia" (Wernicke, 1974), assumed to be a failure of connection between anterior and posterior systems, may be seen in recovering Wernicke's aphasics. It is remarkable in that repetition is claimed to be *more* affected than are other speech functions. We will see that some of the contradictions in the literature relate to the treatment of comprehension, production and repetition as holistic concepts. It turns out that the processing of single syllables proceeds differently from multisyllabic speech, as will become clear in the data presented below.

In general, then, it was assumed that speech input was assimilated, and spontaneous utterances were organized, by the posterior region, whose functions ranged from perception at a phonemic/syllable level, to the processing of meaning. Such input or communicative content was transmitted to the anterior "motor" system, only when needed for the effector side of speaking. Thus, for those who equated speech with linguistic/semantic capacity, the focus of interest was on the complex propositional activity which presumably preceded an utterance. Within this schema, the obvious and frequent errors in production of speech after posterior damage were seen as a consequence, not of a motor organization problem, but of comprehension/semantic deficits.

Although the expressive/receptive dichotomy was found inadequate by various writers on aphasia, e.g., Weisenburg and McBride (1935), no generally acceptable alternative was proposed until the 1960s. Goodglass, Quadfasel, and Timberlake (1964) pointed out that the chief distinguishing feature between Wernicke's and Broca's aphasia was not the contrast between perception and production of speech, but instead, the *type of production error* made in each case. They successfully classified aphasic patients on the basis of one simple measure, phrase length—the number of uninterrupted words in an utterance. This procedure yielded a reliable dichotomy between patients who had very short utterances and those who had utterances more nearly in the normal range. A variation of this method was employed by Benson (1967) in correlating speech fluency with lesion location. He established, as expected, that nonfluent aphasics generally had lesions in the anterior region, and fluent aphasics in the posterior region. After this time, the use of fluency, which formerly had been implicit in many aphasic classifications, became explicit. Rather than serving as an alternative to the older Wernicke/Broca schema, however, it became incorporated into that system by most writers, with the result that the production/comprehension distinction was maintained.

The view that all "higher" functions are vested in the cerebral cortex is a very pervasive one. To some extent, its origins lie in the early detection of the fact that a salient difference between humans and other animals is in the amount of cerebral cortex. Later, when experimental stimulation studies in animals began, the cortex was the most readily accessible and visible structure on which to experiment. However, as far as speech is concerned, the basis for vesting important functions exclusively in the cortex has always been very shaky. Most naturally occurring lesions involve both cortex and underlying white matter, thus interrupting not only cortico-cortical pathways, but also connections between cortex and subcortical nuclei. Even surgical lesions presumably restricted to cortex may, unless great precautions are taken, damage blood vessels which supply areas well beyond the area of excision.

Aside from such negative considerations, however, there is now overwhelming positive evidence (reviewed in Chapter 3) that the thalamus, basal ganglia, and even cerebellum play important roles in speech control, and that such control is asymmetric, as it is for cortical speech systems.

Evidence from stimulation

Most of the data on cortical stimulation come from studies by Penfield and his associates (Penfield & Roberts, 1959; Rasmussen & Milner, 1975), with more recent work carried on by Ojemann (1983). Penfield's data were collected on patients with long-standing epilepsy from early atrophic lesions, usually of the temporal lobe. In order to avoid damage to the critical speech areas in excising the epileptogenic tissue, it was found useful to stimulate the cortex in the awake patient, during speech production, to ascertain whether there was any disturbance to parts of the cortex targeted for removal. Any such areas identified could be avoided in this type of elective surgery. The effects of such stimulation were recorded in detail, and could be classified into four main types—vocalization, hesitation and arrest, articulatory errors, and nonarticulatory errors.

A serious limiting factor in making inferences from stimulation data is the fact that, typically, insufficient information is given concerning how many patients were actually represented in the data points (Penfield & Roberts, 1959). Thus, it is almost impossible to determine whether several points are generated from the same patient or different patients; whether the same patient was in fact stimulated in both anterior and posterior speech areas, or whether limitations of craniotomy size precluded this; whether the small number of patients with speech disturbance from the right hemisphere results from the fact that they were rarely tested for speech effects, and so on. These limitations will be alluded to as they become pertinent throughout this chapter.

Vocalization

Actual vocalization, which was never an intelligible speech sound, but rather a "sustained or interrupted vowel cry" (Penfield & Roberts, 1959), has been obtained from the Rolandic region only, in both left and right hemispheres. This suggests that this area in man forms part of a cortical control system for laryngeal activity. It is interesting to note that vocalization has not been obtained from cortical stimulation in nonhuman primates to date (Robinson, 1967; Jürgens, 1979). Stimulation of the cortical larynx area does however yield vocal fold vibrations in monkeys, and medial frontal lesions affect the ability to master a vocal operant conditioning task (Jürgens, 1989*b*), suggesting the potential for cortical control in nonhumans as well.

Arrest and hesitation

Stimulation which results in interference with speech has been tested while the patient is producing a verbal sequence such as counting, or while the patient is attempting to name an object (Penfield & Roberts, 1959; Rasmussen & Milner, 1975). Simple arrest of speech, and hesitation, which may be considered as a temporary arrest, is obtained from the Rolandic region, again in both left and right hemispheres, in parallel to the production of vocalization.

It is usually claimed that vocalization and arrest from Rolandic stimulation is equally frequent after left- and right-hemisphere stimulation. This is not clearly supported by perusal of the brain mappings (Fig. 4.2) (Penfield & Roberts, 1959), which indicate more points in the left hemisphere which yielded vocalization and arrest. Unfortunately, it is impossible to determine from the data presented, in what *proportion* of left and right stimulations effects occurred, i.e., how many brains or how many stimulations are represented in each sample.

Outside the Rolandic region, arrest of speech appears to be limited to points in the left hemisphere. Rasmussen and Milner (1975) report that arrest produced by stimulation of extra-Rolandic regions (all in the left hemisphere), is different from that produced by Rolandic stimulation, in that the latter also results in inability to move the mouth and tongue during the period that speech is arrested. It is not clear from their report, however, whether this conclusion is based on a systematic comparison between Rolandic and extra-Rolandic regions, or represents a passing observation. A similar effect is implied by the maps presented in Ojemann and Mateer (1979).

Stimulations outside the Rolandic area resulting in arrest or hesitation cluster in what are traditionally considered the anterior and posterior speech areas in the left hemisphere (Penfield & Roberts, 1959). Stimulation of the anterior area produces a higher incidence of simple cessation of speech than does stimulation of the posterior (Fig. 4.3).

Articulatory errors

These are errors in speaking at the syllabic level, and are manifest as slurring, distortion, and repetition of a distorted syllable, all of which involve inaccurate articulation in the production of speech. Repetition of a correctly produced syllable is somewhat more difficult to classify. Slurring, distortion and repetition occur with Rolandic stimulation (Penfield & Roberts, 1959). Slurring (and hesitation) is clearly produced from right Rolandic stimulation as well as from left stimulation, but appears to be considerably less frequent from the right. Again, however, it is not possible to derive the proportional frequency

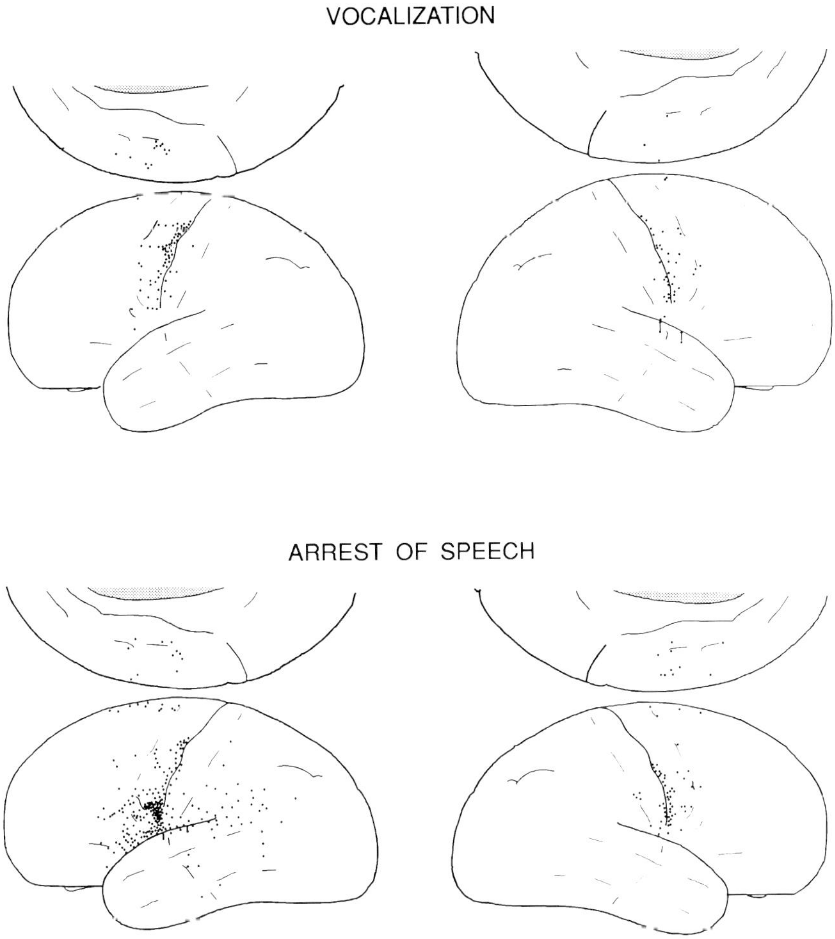

Fig. 4.2 The effects of brain stimulation in left and right hemispheres, on vocalization and arrest of speech. (From Penfield & Roberts, 1959.) Reprinted with permission from Princeton University Press.

because the total sample size, either of patients or stimulations, is not given.

Outside the Rolandic region articulatory effects again occur only from stimulation of the speech areas in the left hemisphere. Hesitation and slurring appear to occur more frequently from anterior stimulation than from posterior stimulation. This does not appear to be true of distortion and repetition (but the same caution applies here as to other frequency statements).

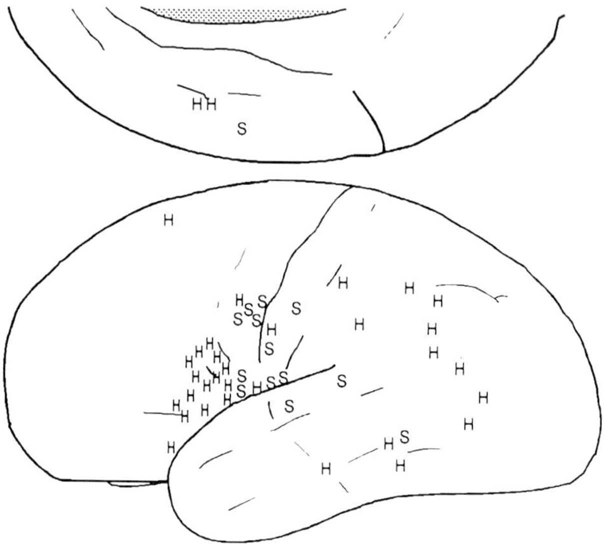

Fig. 4.3 The effects of brain stimulation on hesitation (H) and slurring (S). (From Penfield & Roberts, 1959.)

Nonarticulatory (aphasic) errors

The remaining effects of stimulation on speech which have been studied are confusion of (whole) numbers while counting, misnaming (with or without perseveration), and inability to name with retained ability to speak. All of these responses represent accurate production of some speech, at least at the syllabic level, though the speech may not be correct at the word level, nor relevant to the context. *None* of these effects has been unequivocally elicited by Rolandic stimulation. Outside the Rolandic region, there are no apparent differences between anterior and posterior zones in the frequency of interference of these types. The same appears to be true for Ojemann's (1983) data on naming.

Phoneme discrimination

All of the preceding effects of stimulation have been concerned with production of speech, not with comprehension. Speech perception at the phonemic level has been extensively mapped during cortical stimulation by Mateer (1983). Identification of stop consonants was impaired by stimulation of regions corresponding almost exactly to classical Broca's area, as well as to a larger area in the parieto-temporal region. Thus in the perception of the basic unit of speech, the phoneme, there is clearly a contribution from anterior and posterior speech areas, with no obvious distinction between them.

Summary of stimulation data

It appears that not only voicing, but also some aspects of speech control at a syllabic or phonemic level are mediated to some extent by the left Rolandic region at least, and perhaps also by the right. In the left hemisphere, outside the Rolandic area, interference appears to occur equally often from stimulation of anterior and posterior speech areas, for distortion, slurring, repetition, confusing numbers while counting, misnaming, and inability to name with retained ability to speak. The exception may be in the incidence of arrest (cessation of speech and hesitation), which occurs more often from anterior stimulation. Comprehension of speech at the phoneme level is also affected by anterior or posterior stimulation. These similarities between the effects of anterior and posterior stimulation cannot be due to simple spread of current, since many of the responses are not reproduced by stimulation of Rolandic cortex, which being close to each speech zone, would be susceptible to current spread.

Such findings are not in accord with simple schemas of neural representation of language in which the posterior area receives and comprehends speech, and transmits the verbal message to the anterior zone, which then executes the speech. Producing the correct name of an object appears to be just as affected by anterior as by posterior stimulation, though admittedly there might be different sources of naming difficulty in the two situations, which are not reported in the gross data. The only effect on production which clearly distinguishes anterior and posterior areas is the higher frequency of arrest and hesitation from anterior stimulation. This does indeed suggest that the anterior speech zone has more direct connections with downgoing impulses to speech control musculature, including the basal ganglia systems outlined in Chapter 3. The remainder of the stimulation data, however, suggest that this by no means exhausts or exclusively defines the functions of the anterior region in speaking.

Hesitation and arrest also occur fairly frequently during Rolandic stimulation, even in the right hemisphere. This suggests more functional overlap of the Rolandic cortex with the left anterior non-Rolandic speech area than with the posterior speech area. Whether the Rolandic cortex is an essential relay to the speech musculature, or a normal but dispensable component, cannot be answered from the stimulation data alone.

Evidence from ablations and lesions

Generally, cortical areas presumed to be involved in speech are scrupulously avoided by neurosurgeons. Only in cases where a tumor is situated in such a region, or where a hemorrhagic infarct must be evacuated, is there likely to be removal of a speech area. In such cases there is almost certain to be damage to other cortical regions and to underlying white matter, making it difficult to evaluate the positive findings with reference to precise anatomic localization. Negative findings in such cases are valid, however, and combined consideration of both positive and negative effects can often be instructive. The effects of ablation and pathology will be described under headings corresponding to the locus of damage—Rolandic area, anterior speech zone, and posterior speech zone.

Rolandic region

The pre- and or postcentral gyrus has been surgically excised in cases of focal epilepsy (Penfield & Roberts, 1959; Rasmussen & Milner, 1975). Both studies report that no lasting speech disorders result from removal of the cortical face area of either side, even when both pre- and postcentral face areas are excised. The transient aphasia which is said to be produced by such excisions on the left is not described further. Penfield and Roberts do suggest that face area removals on the left may result in a more persistent and severe "anarthria" than removals on the right, but felt that their series was not large enough to conclude this with certainty. However, we must remember that cortex which has been epileptogenic for many years may no longer be subserving its prepathologic function normally.

Nathan (1947) described several cases of penetrating missile wounds in which the outstanding symptom was "apraxic dysarthria." In all cases there was a speech disorder, characterized in most by a greater difficulty in production of consonants than of vowels. In all six cases, the lesion involved primarily or only the left hemisphere, and minimal extent of the lesion common to all cases was the lower part of the precentral gyrus. Although precise localization was not possible, it appears at least that transient difficulty in tongue and lip control, in both speaking and nonspeech movements, may be caused by lesions to the face area; in all probability such impairment is more likely to occur from damage to the left face area than the right. The general lack of report or comment on such asymmetry may well stem from the prejudice that the "lower level" motor speech functions of the Rolandic region are not likely to be asymmetric, as are the "higher level" functions represented by aphasic disorders. The available data do suggest that the degree of such asymmetry is less than for other cortical areas, but when one recalls that clean *cortical* excisions in other speech areas are rare, even this conclusion must be tentative.

Anterior speech zone

Broca specified an area, damage to which produced "aphemia," or motor aphasia as it is now called, comprising a rather small area in the posterior part of the third frontal convolution (inferior frontal gyrus), involving the pars opercularis and part of the pars triangularis. This corresponds approximately to Brodmann's areas 44 and 45 (Fig. 4.4) (Broca, 1960; Crosby, Humphrey, & Lauer, 1962, p. 514). There has long been serious doubt that Broca's conclusions concerning the critical importance of this circumscribed area were correct, although his general contribution concerning the role of the anterior speech zone has remained valid. Broca's own cases had fairly extensive lesions involving not only the cortex of the inferior frontal region, but invading the white matter underneath, and also the insula. Indeed, in one of his cases, the fluid replacing the brain tissue communicated with the lateral ventricle.

As indicated earlier, surgical excision of even partially healthy cortex in the speech areas is usually avoided. One exception to this is two cases of psychosurgery for psychoses reported by Mettler (1949). In one case Mettler reported excising areas 44 and 45, as well as parts of 46 and 10, *bilaterally*. This patient, a schizophrenic, had been mute before the operation, but began to speak about a month afterward. She apparently spoke in an organized coherent fashion, but had some difficulty with articulation, particularly of consonants, when evaluated again a year after surgery. A detailed account of speech is not given. Since the cortical excision extended beyond the inferior frontal gyrus bilaterally, and may have damaged the foot of the precentral gyrus as well, it is remarkable that the only obvious speech difficulty was related to control of the tongue and lips. A second patient, with area 44 (pars opercularis) removed bilaterally, had no detectable change in speech, which was rather jargonlike before surgery, and remained so with only a temporary remission.

Other cases of Broca's area excisions in the literature involve tumors. Penfield and Roberts (1959) report the removal of Broca's area in one epileptic tumor patient who had, however, a history of speech disturbance associated with seizures, dating from early childhood. Excision of Broca's area resulted in no immediate effect on speech, but the severe transient aphasia a few days later suggested that edema was interfering with other parts of the left hemisphere which subserved some speech function. However, the long history of speech disorder in this individual

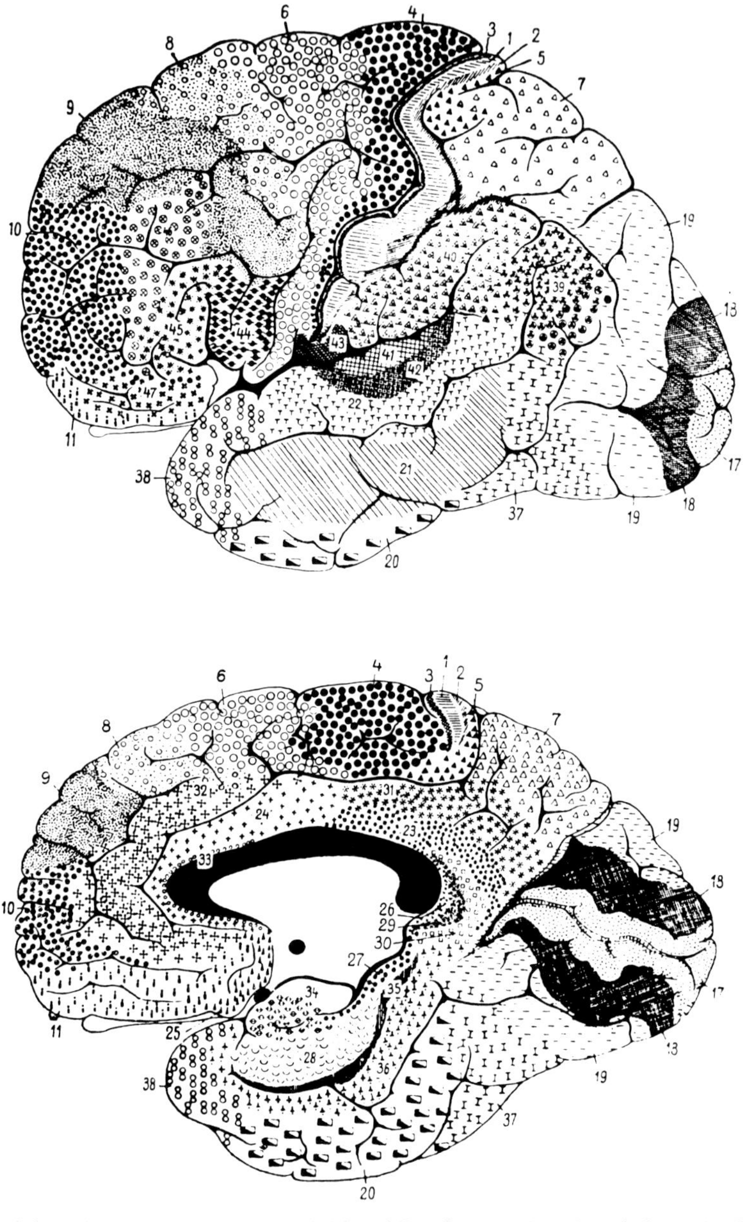

Fig. 4.4 The cytoarchitectonic fields of Brodmann. Reprinted from K. Brodmann, *Vergleichends Lokalisationslehre der Grosshirnrinder*, 1909, p. 131, with permission from J. A. Barth, Leipzig.

may have led to the reorganization of speech, so that the anterior speech area became less critical.

Zangwill (1975) reported on two cases of tumors in the left inferior frontal region. In one case, all of Broca's area was almost certainly removed, and in the other, there was extensive damage to the fibres underneath. In both cases there was a transient speech disorder, but a month later, speech was normal. Zangwill concluded that speech recovery was effected by remaining motor speech systems in the left hemisphere, and that Broca's area is not critical for such function.

Hècaen and Consoli (1973) describe several cases with various etiologies in which damage involved at least Broca's area, and where additional damage was restricted to areas above the Sylvian fissure and anterior to the Rolandic fissure, thus not encroaching on the posterior speech area. (This study is an exception in the literature, in that cases were not selected for symptom, but rather grouped by locus of lesion.) The findings ranged from no significant effect on speech, to severe problems with both production and comprehension. Although the authors claim that "pure" motor aphasia tends to be associated with strictly cortical lesions, and the more mixed aphasia with subcortical damage, the data on location of lesion are not precise enough to warrant such a conclusion, though not incompatible with it.

Pierre Marie (cited by Dejerine) had earlier denied that Broca's area had any function in speech. Dejerine (1913), however, in reviewing his own and other cases in the literature, concluded that lesions of Broca's area did produce impairments in speech, but that if the lesions were restricted to the cortex, such impairments were transitory. Both von Monakow (1914) and Dejerine proposed that the critical area, in the sense that a more than transient disorder occurred after damage, must be larger than areas 44 and 45. Dejerine suggested that the anterior part of the insula might well be part of this system, and von Monakow extended the system to include the Rolandic operculum and the insula. These early suggestions have been supported by recent angiographic and CT scan studies (Cappa and Vignolo, 1983; Mohr, 1976).

Posterior speech zone

The claim that the posterior speech area is primarily devoted to the perception or comprehension of speech is of course attributed to Wernicke (1874, 1911). Wernicke described several cases of sensory aphasia after posterior damage to the first and second left temporal gyri. He states (1911) that "the comprehension of the sound of the words is defective," but "the power of articulate speech is retained." These patients may "make mistakes in the choice of an expression, or employ incorrect or distorted words," which Wernicke attributed to "the lack of a regulating influence of the sensory speech center which determines the choice." Thus was the classical view of distinct motor and sensory speech areas established. Wernicke unquestionably contributed importantly to the early literature on aphasia, but the uncritical acceptance of the idea by later investigators of the extreme separability of motor and sensory speech functions, has been an impediment to further understanding of the details of speech organization.

Nearly all studies on the neural substrate of speech comprehension in the aphasia literature take the form of first categorizing the aphasia as one of a particular type (usually Broca's, Wernicke's, or global—the latter involving both production and comprehension to a significant degree). If correlation with lesion site is attempted, it is then done by looking at the cluster of lesion sites in patients with each type of aphasia. Using such methods, it is typically claimed that speech comprehension (as in Wernicke's aphasia) is affected primarily in posterior lesions. However, the classification of a patient as a Wernicke's aphasic appears to be a complex process, often not very objectively specified, but presupposing a comprehension defect out of proportion to the production problem. In recent years the latter has included the criterion of fluency. Thus the reported dependence of speech comprehension on the posterior region (e.g., Cappa & Vignolo, 1983; Kertesz, 1983) may in fact be reflecting primarily the fluency dimension rather than comprehension.

We can illustrate by comparing two hypothetical aphasic cases *with equivalent comprehension* problems, who might nevertheless be labeled differently by the schemas described above. One has fluent speech, the other nonfluent speech. The former will be designated as a Wernicke's aphasic, the other as a Broca's or global aphasic. The level of speech comprehension ability is not the differentiating feature between these cases, the fluency dimension being the obvious criterion. If the brain lesions in several such cases are viewed together, it is probable that the "Wernicke's" cases will have primarily posterior lesions, and the "Broca's" or "global" cases primarily anterior or generalized damage. However, it would be illogical to conclude from this that speech comprehension depends more on the posterior region, since no independent comparison of comprehension has been done.

This monograph will not employ classifications such as Wernicke's or Broca's aphasia. Instead, we will attempt to systematically describe the speech deficits in patients with pathology in different anatomic systems. It will become apparent that traditional aphasic syndromes do not fit the data very well.

Comparison of anterior and posterior aphasic groups

Aphasia screening tests

Other than Kimura and Watson (1989), there are at present *no studies in the literature in which unselected cases of aphasia are grouped according to lesion sites alone, without reference to aphasic symptoms.* Kimura and Watson presented a major analysis of aphasic subjects, grouped solely on the basis of lesion site, independent of the characteristics of the aphasic disorder. In that analysis, aphasic patients with anterior or posterior lesions did not differ from each other on the Receptive, Expressive, or Modified Token tests (see Chapter 1 for details about the tests). An updated version of the data is presented in Table 4.1, along with scores of patients with right-hemisphere pathology. Though the data for subtests are not shown, anterior and posterior aphasics did not differ on any subtest of the Expressive or Receptive scores either.

Since receptive and expressive function is often claimed to be mediated by posterior and anterior regions, respectively, this rather surprising finding was further analysed by computing the ratio of Receptive to Expressive scores, for each patient. A ratio of 1.00 would indicate equivalent receptive and expressive function, on the tests used, while a ratio substantially less than 1.00 indicates relatively poorer comprehension than production. Although this ratio is higher in aphasics with anterior lesions than those with posterior lesions, this is due almost entirely to one patient with near zero expressive function (who also had very poor scores on Receptive tests). If we consider the anterior group with this one case removed, and also remove one patient from the posterior group who showed a similar but less extreme pattern, then both groups of aphasic patients show essentially equivalent Receptive/Expressive ratios.

Whether these extreme cases are removed from the analyses or not, neither comparison between anterior and posterior groups approaches statistical significance with a *t*-test. Moreover, a Mann–Whitney U-test, comparing ranks rather than absolute scores, does not approach statistical significance either, further confirming that the populations overlap extensively. This can be seen quite readily in Fig. 4.5, where the Receptive/Expressive ratio scores are plotted for all cases. Thus, only one of the anterior-group subjects has a higher score than all of the posterior group, and only three of the posterior group have scores lower than all of the anterior group. Most of the scores in both groups cluster around 1.00. In fact, a higher proportion of the *posterior* cases has receptive scores above the median than is true for anterior cases, just the opposite of what would be predicted from the literature.

Table 4.1 Performance of aphasic patients with left anterior or posterior lesions*

	Left lesions						Right lesions[c]		
	Anterior[a]			Posterior[b]					
	N	$\bar{X}$	(SD)	N	$\bar{X}$	(SD)	N	$\bar{X}$	(SD)
Aphasia tests									
Receptive (/43)	11	34.5	(8.8)	22	34.5	(7.9)	54	42.4	(0.9)
Expressive (/47)	11	36.6	(13.3)	22	37.0	(9.6)	55	46.9	(0.1)
Fluency	11	5.8	(3.6)	21	13.2	(6.1)	10	12.4	(4.3)
Token (/84)	6	60.0	(14.1)	13	62.2	(16.8)	73	82.3	(3.3)
Receptive/Expressive ratio	11	169.5	(239.9)	22	107.5	(33.9)		—	
Without 2 cases	10	97.4	(18.7)	21	101.8	(21.5)		—	
Syllable perception									
Identification (/24)	5	10.4	(5.3)	12	13.3	(5.3)	8	20.1	(1.0)
Same–different (d') (/6)	4	2.4	(1.2)	11	2.7	(1.9)	8	4.4	(1.9)

* Total N = a, 13 (5M, 8F); b, 22 (18M, 4F); c, 73 (43M, 30F).

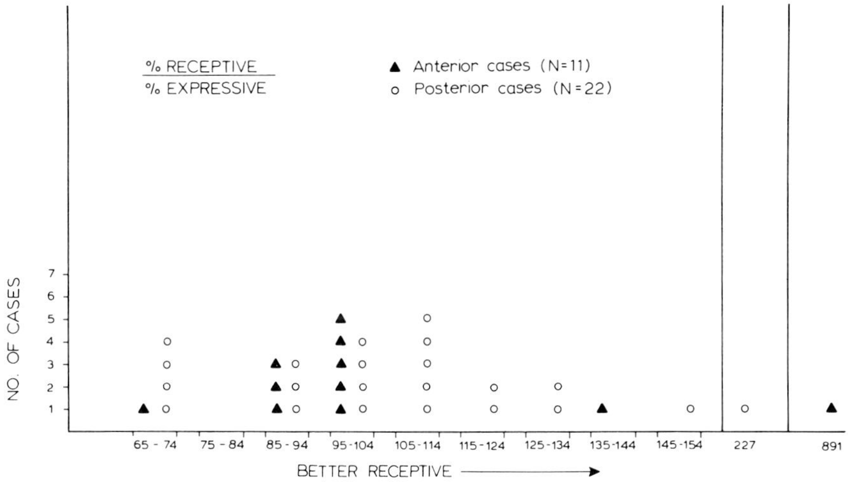

Fig. 4.5 The distribution of aphasic cases with anterior or posterior lesions, on the Receptive/Expressive ratio

On the Fluency measure (the mean number of syllables per utterance in a picture-description task, as outlined in Kimura, 1986), in contrast to the scores on Receptive and Expressive measures, aphasic patients with anterior lesions have significantly lower scores than patients with posterior lesions ($t = 3.70$, df $= 30$, $p < .001$). This would be expected from the literature (Benson, 1967), and indicates that the lack of discrimination on comprehension tests is not due to the fact that our cases are atypical. Figure 4.6, which indicates the fluency scores of all aphasic patients, shows this clear separation of anterior and posterior cases.

Syllable perception

On a speech perception task which requires identification of an individual phoneme/syllable (one of six stop consonants), there is again no obvious difference between the effects of left anterior and posterior lesions (Table 4.1). Mean Identification score of patients with left posterior lesions does not differ significantly from patients with left anterior lesions ($p = .263$), and in any case, the anterior group has the lower score. Both anterior and posterior aphasic groups are significantly inferior to patients with right posterior damage. On a related task in which two successive syllables had only to be discriminated as same or different (d' task), the difference between aphasic subgroups did not approach significance.

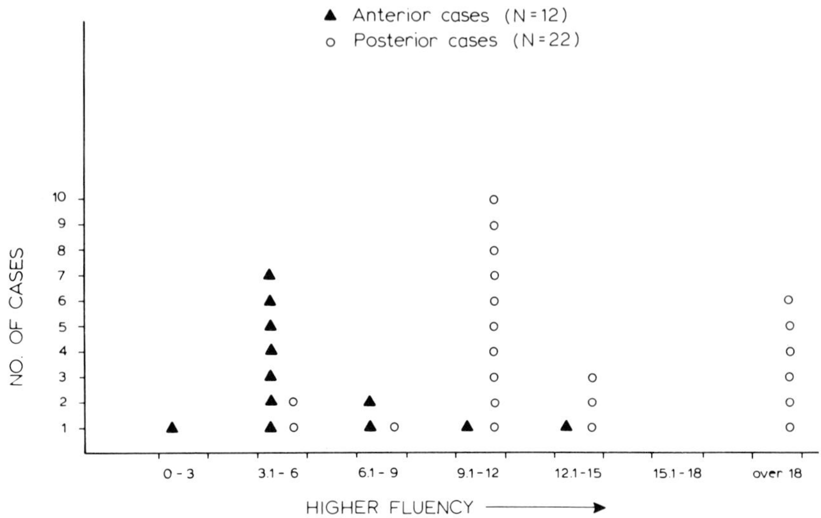

Fig. 4.6 The distribution of aphasic cases with anterior or posterior lesions, on Fluency

The failure to find a difference between anterior and posterior aphasic groups on either discrimination or labeling of isolated stop consonants is consistent with at least two other studies in the literature. In a study by Blumstein, Cooper, Zurif, and Caramazza (1977), grouping of aphasics was not done by locus of lesion, but by Broca's and Wernicke's aphasia. The two groups did not differ on either measure of syllable perception. Basso, Casati, and Vignolo (1977), classified patients as fluent or nonfluent, and found that the nonfluent group had a slightly higher incidence of errors of phoneme identification than did the fluent group.

Speech repetition

Subjects were asked to repeat, immediately after the experimenter uttered them, either individual phonemes/syllables, or familiar phrases. The single sounds ranged from vowels through sibilants, fricatives, liquids and stop consonants. The phrases were simple multisyllabic phrases such as "much food," "saves time," scored for the number of individual phonemes correctly reproduced. As Fig. 4.7 indicates, aphasic patients with anterior lesions have significant difficulty with the reproduction of single speech sounds. This would perhaps be predicted from the fact that anterior lesions often result in articulatory problems (Blumstein and coworkers, 1977; Katz, 1988; Ziegler and von Cramon, 1989). However, what is surprising is their relatively good repetition

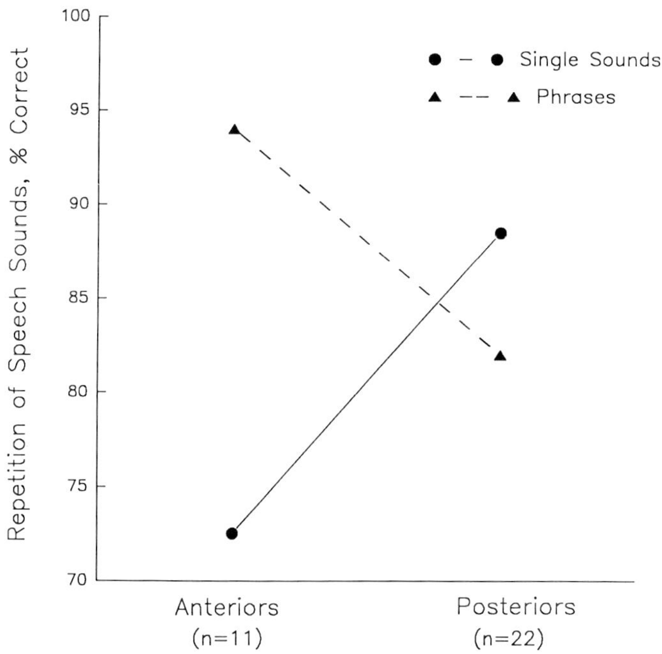

Fig. 4.7 Repetition of speech sounds in aphasic cases with anterior or posterior lesions.

of connected speech in the form of phrases. They are obviously able to circumvent their impairment in the reproduction of the elements of speech, when presented with several elements in a row.

In contrast, aphasic patients with posterior lesions have minor difficulties with single speech sounds, but are significantly impaired, relative to the anterior group, in the reproduction of phrases. There is a significant task × locus interaction ($F = 5.68$, df $= 1, 30$, $p < .03$), and the difference between the two groups is significant for both single sounds ($p < .04$) and phrases ($p < .03$).

An alternative schema

The data suggest that a significant differentiating factor in the functions of anterior and posterior speech areas is the level of control of the speech unit. The anterior region appears to be paramount for mediating production of speech at the phonemic/syllabic level, while the posterior area is less critical at this phase. Conversely, the posterior region is critical for mediating speech production at the multisyllabic level, when the units must be organized into words, phrases, etc.

Surprisingly, a defective single-syllable (anterior) system can be circumvented, under circumstances of simple repetition, when multisyllabic speech is required. This suggests that the reproduction of multisyllabic speech need not proceed syllable-by-syllable, but presumably can under some circumstances short-circuit the anterior syllabic system. Data presented in the next section suggest that the temporal lobe is a critical component of a system for repetition of word-level speech.

On the receptive side also, Basso and coworkers (1977) suggested that multisyllabic or word-level comprehension is not necessarily predicted by defects at the phonemic level. Thus a deficit in discriminating phonemes need not be a severe handicap when listening to connected speech. This may be due in part to the fact that context and redundancy in speech provide cues which reduce the necessity for a phoneme-by-phoneme analysis, but there may also be other bypassing mechanisms available.

Subdivisions within the posterior region

Within the limitations of sample size, and the determination of lesion location, no functional subdivisions could be made within the left anterior region. With increased sample sizes, such differentiation might yet occur. In the posterior region, patterns of impairment emerged which were discriminably different between patients whose damage was restricted primarily to the temporal lobe, or primarily to the parietal lobe. There were nine cases with primarily temporal and six with primarily parietal damage. The remaining seven cases with posterior lesions had damage which was more extensive and cut across at least two lobar divisions. The data for all three groups—anterior, temporal, and parietal—are shown in Table 4.2. (Note that data for anterior cases are identical to Table 4.1.)

It does not appear that there are any striking differences on the aphasia screening tests, although with the greatly reduced sample sizes, such statements must be tentative. Data for Syllable Perception are not shown for the parietal group, because only two cases with parietal damage were tested. However, on the reproduction of unisyllabic and multisyllabic speech (single sounds and phrases), a difference in pattern does appear (Fig. 4.8, updated from Kimura & Watson, 1989). Patients with temporal-lobe damage have minimal difficulty in repeating back single speech sounds, but have great difficulty with multisyllabic phrases. Patients with parietal-lobe damage are better able to repeat back phrases than temporal-lesioned patients.

Thus a 2 × 3 (task by locus) analysis of variance on the data depicted in Fig. 4.8 yielded a significant locus by task interaction ($F = 5.94$,

Table 4.2 Performance of aphasic patients with primarily anterior, temporal, or parietal lesions*

	Anterior[a]			Temporal[b]			Parietal[c]		
Aphasic screening tests	N	$\bar{X}$	(SD)	N	$\bar{X}$	(SD)	N	$\bar{X}$	(SD)
Receptive (/43)	11	34.5	(8.8)	9	37.2	(6.3)	6	30.3	(10.2)
Expressive (/47)	11	36.6	(13.3)	9	37.6	(9.1)	6	35.3	(12.6)
Ratio Expressive/Receptive	11	169.5	(239.9)	9	117.6	(45.7)	6	97.5	(26.4)
(without extreme cases)	10	97.4	(18.7)	8	103.9	(21.5)	6	97.5	(26.4)
Fluency	11	5.8	(3.6)	8	13.5	(7.3)	6	11.2	(4.9)
Token test (/84)	6	60.0	(14.1)	5	73.0	(8.0)	4	60.5	(13.2)
Syllable identification (/24)	5	10.4	(5.3)	5	15.6	(6.3)	—	—	—

* Total N = a, 13 (5M, 8F); b, (6M, 3F); c, 6 (6M, 0F).

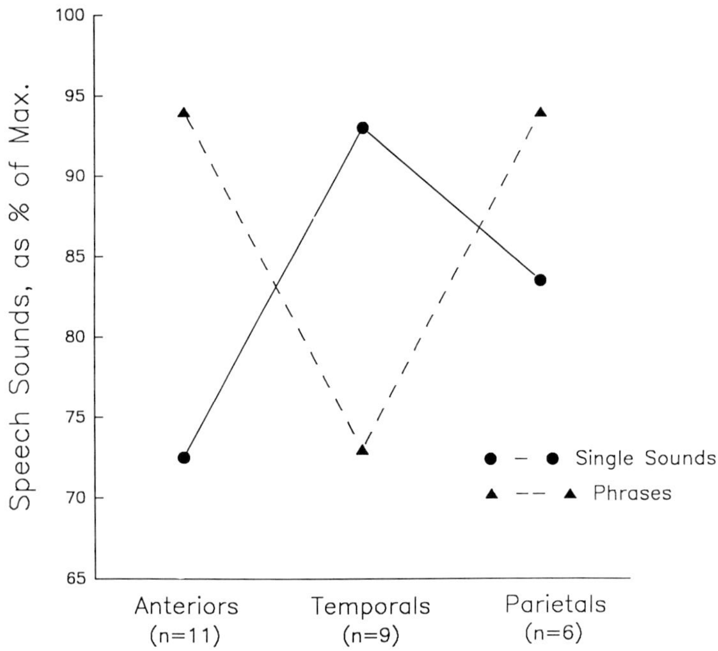

Fig. 4.8 Repetition of speech sounds in aphasic cases with anterior, temporal, or parietal lesions.

df = 2, 22, $p < .01$). Subsequent one-tailed *t*-tests yielded the following *p* levels, on Single Speech—anterior vs. temporal: $p < .01$; anterior vs. parietal: $p < .10$; temporal vs. parietal: $p < .05$; on Phrases—anterior vs. temporal: $p < .04$; anterior vs. parietal: $p < .50$; temporal vs. parietal: $p < .05$. On multisyllabic speech, both parietal and anterior lesions cause less impairment than do temporal lesions.

The difficulty which patients with temporal-lobe damage experience in repeating back multisyllabic speech does not appear to be reducible to speech-comprehension problems. Their scores on the Receptive part of the aphasia screening tests are, if anything, higher than other aphasic groups (Table 4.2). The same is true of the Token test, a very demanding test of speech perception, and of Syllable Perception, though the sample sizes on these tests are quite small. The relatively good performance on the Token test also seems to argue against the possibility of a verbal short-term memory deficit (Warrington, Logue, & Pratt, 1971) as an explanation for the poor repetition. The Token test requires the subject to carry out sequential verbal commands directed to colored chips of various shapes and sizes, and is thus quite demanding of short term memory span. The mean score of temporal-lobe aphasics (73.0,

Table 4.2), is at the top end of the aphasic range, near the cutoff score of 75 for aphasic classification (Kimura, 1986). It appears that where the speech input needs only to be encoded into a concrete referent, this can be achieved relatively well after temporal-lobe damage.

What appears to be impaired in temporal-lobe aphasics is the ability to repeat back words, i.e., some type of verbal–echolalic function. This bears a certain similarity to what has been called "conduction aphasia" (relatively good comprehension and fluency with impaired repetition), said to arise from the lesions of the temporo-parietal region (e.g., Damasio & Damasio, 1980, 1983). However, it should be noted that our temporal-lobe damaged aphasics can repeat back single sounds quite well. It is on multisyllabic material that they have greatest difficulty. This is probably not due simply to the greater ease of repeating back single syllables, since the anterior group, by contrast, is more impaired on the single than the multiple task. No information is available in the literature on the ability of "conduction aphasics" to repeat back isolated sounds, but the label implies that all repetition should be affected.

Our data suggest that the temporal speech area has some special function in organizing speech output in word units, or connected-speech units of some kind, perhaps specifically under auditory control. Thus the second (multisyllabic) level of speech control may further comprise two separable systems, the temporal and parietal, which contribute primarily verbal–acoustic and motor programming functions, respectively. We will return to this comparison between temporal and parietal contributions to speech in Chapter 5, which discusses the relation between oral-movement control and speech.

Summary

Aphasic patients with damage restricted to the anterior or posterior speech zones, respectively, do not differ on various tasks of speech perception and comprehension. They do differ on measures of speech fluency, and on the type of speech-repetition task most affected. Aphasic patients with anterior lesions have reduced fluency and show impairment in repeating back isolated speech sounds or syllables, though multisyllabic speech can be repeated relatively well. Aphasic patients with posterior lesions, in contrast, have fluent speech and tend to have little difficulty with repetition of isolated syllables. However, those cases with primarily temporal-lobe damage tend to have greater difficulty in repeating back multisyllabic speech.

It appears that anterior and posterior speech systems represent two levels of speech control, unisyllabic and multisyllabic, respectively. Within the multisyllabic level, however, there are differences between temporal and parietal regions, the former contributing a verbal echolalic component.

5. Oral movement control and speech

Central nervous system disorders in the control of the oral musculature in humans have been reported in close association with aphasia and are typically a consequence of left-hemisphere pathology. Impairment in the performance of oral movements, called oral apraxia, is more frequently reported in particular kinds of speech disorders. Thus aphasias labeled "motor," "Broca's" (DeRenzi, Pieczuro, & Vignolo, 1966), articulatory (LaPointe & Wertz, 1974), and "nonfluent" (Mateer & Kimura, 1977), all are likely to have an associated oral apraxia. They are also characterized by halting laborious speech or short utterances, suggesting a motor coordination problem. This is in contrast to aphasias labeled "Wernicke's" or "fluent" (see Chapter 4).

Typically, oral movement function has been examined with relatively simple single movements, such as protruding the tongue, whistling, puffing the cheeks, and so on (deRenzi & coworkers, 1966; Poeck & Kerschensteiner, 1975). Difficulties in the production of such single oral movements are more common after damage to the left anterior region of the brain than after posterior damage, consistent with their close association with Broca's and/or nonfluent aphasia (Tognola & Vignolo, 1980; Kimura, 1982). The infrequency of oral-movement defects after posterior lesions or in fluent aphasia has sometimes been cited as evidence that the posterior speech area, in contrast to the anterior, is involved primarily in linguistic or speech-specific functions (see Geschwind, 1972, 1979).

We have argued that if nonverbal oral-movement control parallels oral-movement control in speech, we would expect the posterior region to operate at a level more complex than a single oral movement. Fluent aphasia, resulting from a posterior lesion, does not typically result in speech errors at the articulatory single-syllable level, but rather when coordinating several units into connected speech (Mateer & Kimura, 1977; Kimura, 1982; Kimura & Watson, 1989). One might therefore expect that any analogous oral-movement defect would be detectable primarily when more than one movement is to be produced. To test this suggestion, Mateer and Kimura presented not only single oral movements for imitation, of the kind used by most investigators (protrude tongue, open mouth, and so on), but also three of these movements in sequence. As predicted, fluent aphasics had no difficulty in imitating one oral movement, but they were impaired in copying the multiple oral movements. Of course, nonfluent aphasics, who have difficulty reproducing even a single oral movement, also have difficulty with multiple movements.

The degree to which speech and nonspeech oral-movement defects co-occur should be indicative of the necessity for postulating divergent or additional control mechanisms not common to both. This chapter will investigate that relationship, and will examine briefly the relation between oral-movement control and manual-movement control

Reproduction of oral movements

Two tasks were presented live by the experimenter for immediate imitation by the patient (see Chapter 1 for details). The first consisted of a series of relatively simple single movements, presented one at a time for immediate reproduction. Examples are lateralizing the tongue (any direction), blowing, chattering teeth, and so on. In the second or multiple-movements task, a series of three different oral movements were presented on each trial, and the patient was required to imitate all three movements after the last one was presented. It was expected that production of the single movements would be affected by anterior pathology, but that posterior damage would affect only the multiple oral movements.

Table 5.1 presents an overview of performance on both single-oral and multiple-oral movement tasks, across several patient groups with left or right lesions localized to the anterior, central, or posterior sectors of the brain (Kimura & Watson, 1989). Some data on age-matched normal subjects were also available on the single oral movements task.

Table 5.1 Single-oral and multiple-oral movement scores

	Left lesions			Right lesions			Normals		
Task	*N*	Score	(SD)	*N*	Score	(SD)	*N*	Score	(SD)
Single oral (/17)									
Anterior	29	14.2	(3.9)	21	16.1	(1.0)	15	16.9	(0.35)
Central	22	15.7	(1.5)	19	16.6	(.7)			
Posterior	69	15.9	(1.6)	34	16.2	(1.1)			
Multiple oral (/9)									
Anterior	21	5.3	(2.9)	17	6.7	(1.8)		—	
Central	15	7.1	(1.0)	11	7.6	(1.3)			
Posterior	61	5.7	(2.2)	22	7.3	(1.4)			

Table 5.2 Single- and multiple-oral movements in aphasic patients with left anterior or posterior lesions

	Single oral (/17)			Multiple oral (/9)		
Locus of lesion	*N*	Score	(SD)	*N*	Score	(SD)
Anterior	12	11.1	(4.4)	7	2.1	(2.3)
Posterior	22	15.4	(1.9)	21	3.9	(2.1)

Patients are initially included here, whether or not they are aphasic, to get an unbiased view of the contribution of a particular anatomic system to these tasks. (The number of aphasic subjects in each group is shown in Table 5.2.)

For single oral movements, a 2 × 3 (side × locus) analysis of variance yielded a significant effect of side ($F = 7.667$, df = 1, 181, $p < .01$), as well as of locus ($F = 3.958$, df = 2, 181, $p = .02$). The interaction between side and locus is not significant. When a priori *t*-tests were used to compare the left anterior group with the other five groups, the differences were significant in each case beyond the .01 level. Thus the only group which is unequivocally impaired in reproducing single oral movements is the left anterior group.

Of patient groups with lesions of comparable locus on the two sides, in addition to the two anterior groups, those with left and right *central* lesions also differ significantly from each other ($p < .02$). Since the mean age, etiology (primarily tumors), and extent of damage are quite similar in these two groups, it appears that there is a mild impairment in producing single oral movements after left central damage as well, in agreement with a report by Nathan (1947). Nevertheless, the left central group performs significantly better than the left anterior.

On multiple-oral movements in an equivalent group of patients, the analysis of variance again yielded a highly significant effect of side ($F = 14.244$, df = 1, 134, $p < .001$), with the left-damaged groups the more impaired. There is also a significant effect of locus ($F = 3.716$, df = 2, 134, $p < .03$), but as expected on this task, the left anterior and posterior groups do not differ from each other. The superior performance of the left central group largely reflects the absence of aphasics in this group. There is no significant difference between left and right central groups on multiple oral movements, though the trend is the same as for single movements.

Even in aphasic patients (Table 5.2), those with posterior lesions usually manage to achieve a score of 15 out of 17 on single oral movements, in contrast to poor performance by aphasic patients with anterior lesions ($t = 2.81$, df corrected for heterogeneous variances = 11.9, $p < .02$). On multiple oral movements, however, the two aphasic groups do not differ significantly ($t = 1.38$, df = 24, $p = 179$, n.s.). Both are clearly impaired, relative to right-damaged groups.

Thus, these data show that the left anterior region is paramount for the reproduction of single oral movements, the posterior region being apparently quite dispensable in this regard. For accurate reproduction of multiple oral movements, however, the posterior region must be intact. It appears therefore to play a role in selecting movements, which becomes evident only when more than one movement is required. However, a damaged anterior system is also a limiting factor in the reproduction of multiple movements. These findings are essentially confirmed by cortical stimulation studies (Ojemann, 1983), where disruption of single (repeated) oral movements is achieved only by anterior stimulation. Disruption of several sequential oral movements is achieved by anterior or posterior stimulation.

Speeded articulation tasks

Performance on the oral movement tasks showed a remarkably similar pattern of performance across lesion groups, to a demanding speech-articulation task. The first part of the articulation task required the rapid repetition of a single consonant–vowel syllable (first trial "ba," second trial "ga") for 5 sec. The score was the mean number of such repetitions correctly repeated in 5 sec. In the second part of the task, the required sequence was "ba-da-ga," thus a changing series of syllables. Again the score was the mean number of correct syllables over two such trials (Mateer & Kimura, 1977; Kimura, 1986).

Table 5.3 shows the data for left- and right-damaged patients with anterior, central, or posterior lesions (Kimura & Watson, 1989). Data were also available for age-matched normal subjects. A 2 × 3 (side × locus) analysis of variance for the data on single syllable repetition yielded only a significant locus effect ($F = 4.024$, df = 2, 68, $p < .02$). This reflects the fact that the left anterior group was significantly inferior to every other group (p ranged from .05 to .001). This is the same pattern as was observed for performance on the single oral movements.

On multi-syllabic speeded repetition, both the left anterior and left posterior groups were significantly impaired, just as they are on multiple oral movements. This is reflected in a significant effect of side ($F = 4.869$, df = 1, 68, $p < .03$), but not of locus. Both groups are also significantly inferior to the normal group.

Fewer aphasic patients were given this task than was the case for the nonverbal oral movements tasks, since it was included later in our

Table 5.3 Speeded articulation (syllables per 5 sec)

	Left lesions			Right lesions			Normals		
Task	*N*	Score	(SD)	*N*	Score	(SD)	*N*	Score	(SD)
Single ("ba/ga")									
Anterior	10	21.9	(3.9)	9	29.4	(7.3)	17	28.7	(3.6)
Central	8	28.5	(5.0)	7	29.8	(5.2)			
Posterior	33	29.4	(4.6)	8	29.3	(4.3)			
Multiple ("ba-da-ga")									
Anterior	10	18.5	(10.6)	9	26.0	(7.3)	17	30.4	(6.2)
Central	8	29.5	(5.1)	7	26.3	(5.4)			
Posterior	33	22.8	(11.8)	8	31.9	(4.8)			

Table 5.4 Speeded articulation in aphasic patients with left anterior or posterior lesions

	Single ("ba/ga")			Multiple ("ba-da-ga")		
Locus	*N*	Score	(SD)	*N*	Score	(SD)
Anterior	3	17.2	(15.8)	3	6.0	(10.4)
Posterior	10	28.9	(3.8)	10	13.2	(15.0)

series of patients. However, even for the small group of aphasic cases with anterior or posterior lesions (Table 5.4), a Mann–Whitney *U*-test yielded a difference between groups on the single repetition task at the .05 level (one tailed). What is very clear is that the 10 aphasic patients with posterior pathology have no difficulty in performing this task, as judged by the comparison with right-damaged cases and normal subjects in Table 5.3.

On multisyllabic speeded repetition ("ba-da-ga"), both groups of aphasic patients were impaired, as they were on multiple oral movements. It should be noted that the difficulty which posteriorly damaged aphasic patients experienced in "ba-da-ga" repetition was not due simply to the speeded nature of the task. First, speeded repetition of a single syllable was unaffected, indicating that simply increasing the demands on articulation had no effect. Moreover, most such patients, even if ultimately able to repeat the three syllables correctly, required more than one trial even in the unspeeded practise phase of the task.

Correlations between speech and nonspeech tasks

In Chapter 4 we noted that aphasics with anterior lesions were impaired in repeating back a single phoneme or syllable, while those with posterior lesions had relatively little difficulty on that task. This of course parallels the findings above for rapid repetition of a syllable, and for immediate reproduction of a single oral movement.

However, on simple unspeeded reproduction of *phrases,* aphasics with anterior lesions actually performed better than they did on reproducing single sounds, an apparently anomalous finding. They also performed better than aphasics with posterior lesions, unlike the pattern for "ba-da-ga" or multiple oral movements. It appears that, in repetition of connected speech which does not stress articulation mechanisms, the impediment of an anterior lesion can be overcome or circumvented in some way, as long as the posterior region is intact. We will discuss the possible circumventing system later in this chapter.

Taken together, the findings suggest a tight association among the neural systems underlying all "single" oral movements, whether these be speech movements or not, and whether they be simply repeated back, or must be articulated rapidly. If so, we should see high correlations between speech and nonspeech movements, across a large sample of patients with left-hemisphere pathology. Table 5.5 shows such

Table 5.5 Correlations of oral movement tasks with single-syllable speech tasks

	Single speech reproduction		Speeded speech ("ba/ga")	
Group	*r*	(*N*)	*r*	(*N*)
All left lesions				
Single oral	.896	(192)	.782	(104)
Multiple oral	.634	(133)	.470	(104)
All aphasics				
Single oral	.882	(100)	.813	(40)
Multiple oral	.496	(76)	.394*	(38)

* $p < .000$ in all cases except this ($p = .007$).

correlations, both for single oral movements and for multiple oral movements.

The correlations between single oral movement reproduction and simple unspeeded reproduction of a speech sound are extremely high ($r = .90$), despite the fact that the two tasks are presented quite differently, one being a visual presentation, and one an auditory presentation. In fact, a correlation of this magnitude, even uncorrected for limitations of reliability, suggests that, throughout most of the system, the two functions overlap almost completely. Moreover, the correlations with "ba/ga" are also very high, and the difference between single oral/single speech and single oral/speeded speech is not significant in any case. The slightly lower correlations for "ba/ga" may simply reflect a smaller sample size in the latter case.

The impressively high correlations between single speech and non-speech movements appear to be at variance with previous suggestions that motor aphasia and oral apraxia can be dissociated (DeRenzi & coworkers, 1966; Poeck & Kerschensteiner, 1975; Tognola & Vignolo, 1980; Heilman, Rothi, & Kertesz, 1983). There are a number of reasons why this dissociation may be seen. One suggestion has been that, although both functions depend on the same system, one may be less sensitive to damage to the region in question than the other (deRenzi & coworkers, 1966).

A more probable explanation of the reported dissociations, however, relates to problems of measurement. First, oral apraxia is typically measured by requiring a very small sample of oral movements, often highly practised, and thus not maximally sensitive to a movement defect. In contrast, the measures of aphasia, although variable from study to study, are always much more extensive. The fewer items a test contains, of course, the less reliable will be the measure. Therefore, unless the oral apraxia scale has at least 10 items, varying in difficulty, the actual measure of oral praxis is unlikely to be ideal. Second, the procedure of using cutoff scores (see Chapter 1), and comparing concordant and nonconcordant classifications, tends to exaggerate dissociations. Often the nonconcordant classifications emanate from scores which are actually quite near the cutoff of one class or the other. Correlations are thus more likely to give a truer picture of the relationship between two variables.

We can illustrate this with some details from the data. The correlation between single speech reproduction and single oral movement reproduction is .90, as already noted (Table 5.5). If we use the scores of patients with right-hemisphere lesions to decide on cutoff scores to indicate impairment on these tasks, as is typically done, we would conclude that a score of less than 18 out of 20 on single speech, and of less than 14 out of 17 on single oral movements is defective.

Table 5.6 "Dissociations" between phoneme and single oral movement reproduction

Cutoff scores yielding less than 10% "impaired" in patients with right-hemisphere damage:

Single oral movements—below 14 (max. = 17)
Single phonemes —below 18 (max. = 20)

In 192 patients with left-hemisphere pathology, given both tasks:

above cutoff on both —104
below cutoff on both— 62
discrepant — 26 ($13\frac{1}{2}\%$)

Of 26 "discrepant", only 3 are more than 2 points from cutoff on either task (1.6% of 192 cases)

Scanning the 192 cases (Table 5.6) making up this correlation, we find 104 who are above the cutoff on both tasks, 62 who are below the cutoff on both, and 26 who are below the cutoff on one, but above it on the other task. The latter are not all "impaired" or "spared" on the same task. This would seem to indicate a 13% discordancy rate (26/192), suggesting that the performance of single oral movements and single speech sounds can be dissociated with this frequency. However, when we examine these 26 cases, we find that the scores in nearly every case hover around the cutoff level on one test or the other. The number of cases with widely discrepant scores on the two tests is only 3, or less than 2%, a number which might occur by chance. That is, variations in the state of attention or of fatigue from one test to another might well give rise to a discrepancy of this frequency. Clearly, using the scores of an intact group to decide on cutoffs, in combination with imperfect measures, may give rise to *apparent* dissociations of this type. This is not, of course, a problem unique to oral apraxia.

Mouth asymmetry for speech and nonspeech tasks

Further evidence that speech and nonspeech movements are subserved by the same system comes from studies on mouth asymmetry in normal persons. Graves, Goodglass, and Landis (1982) reported that when people speak, the right side of the mouth opens wider than the left. They also reported that the effect was specific to speech (Graves & Landis, 1985), and interpreted this finding as another reflection of the left hemisphere's control of speech.

Subsequent studies, however, demonstrated that the right-bias asymmetry was present for nonspeech movements as well (Wolf & Goodale, 1987). Subjects were required, for the speech task, either to repeat a single syllable over and over (as in the speeded repetition described above), or to repeat changing syllables. The nonverbal mouth movements consisted of parallel tasks of either performing a single oral movement over and over (e.g., open mouth), or repeating several movements in a row (open mouth, blow, close mouth, and so on). The right bias was just as strong for nonspeech movements as for speech tasks, and this held for both single and multiple movements.

Thus to the degree that mouth asymmetry reflects hemispheric asymmetry, it appears that the left hemisphere is equally necessary for control of speaking and nonspeaking movements. We shall see in Chapters 6 and 8 that the same holds true for manual movements, i.e., that both linguistic and nonlinguistic movements are dependent on this hemisphere for accurate programming. Within the left hemisphere, of course, there are differential contributions from different anatomic systems, as we shall see at the end of this chapter.

Jürgens (1989*c*) reviews evidence that in the monkey, the anterior cingulate region is critical for the initiation of vocalization, although it does not determine the content of such vocalization. Jürgens and vonCramon (1982) reported on a human case of mutism associated with bilateral damage to the anterior cingulate region and left supplementary motor region. The chief characteristic of speech when it returned, after a phase of whispering, was the loss of appropriate intonation. Neither in this case, nor in others in the literature is there information on whether nonvocal oral movements are affected. We did see a case of akinetic mutism[1] in whom we were able to evaluate both speech and nonspeech oral movements.

A case of mutism

The 29-year-old woman was well until she developed a right hemiplegia, right hemianopsia and questionable global aphasia. When admitted to the local hospital, she was mute and unresponsive, occasionally following commands correctly, but also appearing easily distracted. The period of muteness lasted fully a month, and was followed by variable output in speech, with the patient generally extremely reluctant to talk, though eventually able to utter coherent phrases and sentences when she finally did speak. The computed tomography and magnetic resonance imaging scans performed about 6 weeks after her stroke showed not only the expected pathology in the left hemisphere in basal ganglia and medial frontal regions (including supplementary motor), but also a right medial frontal and parasagittal infarct, extending into the anterior cingulate.

The patient was tested fairly extensively, but the discussion will concentrate on the parallel between the speaking and oral movement deficits. She was minimally aphasic, as measured on the usual aphasia screening tests (see Chapter 4), but her spontaneous naming was extremely slow. On a test of speeded picture-naming she averaged 31.3 sec to name 10 familiar objects, compared to the average of *aphasic* patients of 17.6 sec (SD = 6.8) and about 6 sec for non-aphasics (Kimura, Interference Naming test, 1986). Naming of colours was also slower than the mean for aphasics. She also managed to generate only one word beginning with the letter "d" in 60 sec. Her difficulties were seen primarily in spontaneous speech, repetition of phrases and multi-syllabic words being near normal.

When initially requested to imitate oral movements she was completely unwilling or unable to imitate any except the most common, such as opening the mouth or sticking out the tongue, and even here she had inordinately long latencies. Over the course of several days' presentation of these same movements, she eventually completed 11 of the 17, though with apparent reluctance and difficulty and consistently long latency. This is the same score as the mean of aphasic patients with left anterior lesions (Table 5.2), but such patients make prompt attempts at copying. When presented with more than one oral movement, she was completely unable to copy any, though in later stages of the testing she could sometimes describe one of the movements. She also could not produce oral movements to command.

These difficulties with oral movements and with speech contrasted sharply with her prompt and accurate copying of manual movements (tests described in Chapter 6), indicating that she did not have any generalized problem in processing movements presented to her. Similarly, she was only slightly below average on constructional tasks, and performed very well on certain other tests, including a spatial rotation test involving identification of hands (by pointing).

It thus appears that the akinetic mutism generally attributed to damage to the anterior cingulate region may not involve only vocalization, but may extend to other kinds of oral movements. No other cases have been examined from this point of view, but the symptoms in the case just described, point up again the potentially close association between the mechanisms controlling speech and nonspeech movements. While these certainly may diverge, as suggested below for temporal- and parietal-lobe contributions, for most phases of control they appear to overlap extensively.

Relations among oral and manual tasks

Correlations of all speech-task scores with multiple oral movements are significantly lower than with single oral movements (the difference between correlations is significant at beyond the $p < .01$ level in all four comparisons, Table 5.5). If the multiple oral task were simply a more difficult form of the single oral, just the opposite might be expected. Correlations between single and multiple oral tasks (Table 5.7) also

Table 5.7 Correlations* among oral and manual tasks

	Single oral		Manual movements	
	N	*r*	*N*	*r*
All patients with left-hemisphere lesions				
Multiple oral	193	.645	193	.670
Single oral	—	—	244	.603
Aphasic patients only				
Multiple oral	80	.542	79	.566
Single oral	—	—	98	.503

* All correlations are significant beyond .01 level.

indicate that, while the two tasks are significantly related, they are not tightly associated.

As Table 5.7 shows, the multiple oral task is at least as highly correlated with *manual* movements as with single oral movements. (The manual task requires the copying of unfamiliar hand-and-arm movements and has proved quite sensitive to manual apraxia.) This finding confirms the suggestion made earlier in this chapter that adequate performance of multiple oral movements requires the participation of another system in addition to the left anterior system responsible for production of single movements. The system responsible for controlling multiple oral and manual movements must lie outside the single-oral movement system.

Developmental data reported by Ramsay (1980, 1984) on the coincidence of babbling and hand preference in infants also supports the suggestion that some aspects of oral and manual control tap into the same system. The onset of unimanual hand preference coincided with the onset of duplicated syllable babbling, whereas bimanual hand preference coincided with nonduplicated (multisyllabic) babbling. He attributed the findings to a manifestation of different stages of development of the left hemisphere.

Comparison of temporal and parietal contributions

In Chapter 4 it was suggested that temporal- and parietal-lobe systems may contribute somewhat different controlling functions to speech. The temporal-lobe system appeared to be more essential for echoic reproduction of connected speech, detectable in repeating back multisyllabic phrases. Yet when we examine the speeded articulation of changing syllables ("ba-da-ga"), just the reverse pattern is obtained, with parietal-lesioned aphasics the more impaired. The sample sizes on the latter task were unfortunately quite small (four temporal and three parietal aphasics). Both groups achieved normal scores on speeded repetition of single syllables ("ba/ga"), but on "ba-da-ga" the parietal-lobe aphasics achieved a mean of only 1.5 syllables in 5 sec (near zero performance), while the temporal-lobe aphasics achieved 19.5. The deficit in the parietal group was not due only to the speed demands of the task, since repeating three different syllables twice in a row, unspeeded, presented difficulties.

These preliminary rapid-articulation data suggest that we might expect the two groups to differ in a parallel manner in reproducing nonspeech oral or manual movements. That is, left parietal damage might be expected to result in greater difficulty with such multiple movements than would occur after left temporal damage. Manual praxis will be discussed in detail in Chapter 6, but we consider it briefly here because it helps elucidate the functional specialization between these two posterior regions in oral-movement control. Table 5.8 shows the mean scores for three aphasic subgroups on oral and manual movement tasks.

Again on single oral movements, both the posterior groups perform quite well, and there is no trace of a difference between them. On multiple oral movements, however, there is a trend for temporal-lobe aphasics to be less impaired than parietal-lobe aphasics ($t = 2.09$, df = 13, $p < .07$). The F ratio across all three groups also shows such a trend ($F = 2.68$, df = 2, 18, $p < .10$). On copying manual movements, where overall sample sizes are slightly larger, there was a significant overall effect of group ($p < .02$), the temporal group having significantly higher scores than the anterior ($p < .03$) or the parietal ($p < .01$)

Table 5.8 Single-oral and multiple-oral movements in aphasic patients with localized lesions

	Single oral (/17)			Multiple oral (/9)			Manual movements (/24)		
Locus	*N*	Mean	(SD)	*N*	Mean	(SD)	*N*	Mean	(SD)
Anterior	12	11.1	(4.4)	7	2.1	(2.3)	12	10.0	(5.5)
Temporal	9	15.9	(1.5)	8	4.8	(2.7)	8	15.9	(5.9)
Parietal	6	15.7	(1.5)	6	3.3	(1.0)	6	7.3	(2.8)

groups, but the latter two did not differ. Thus the parietal region appears to contribute more to the organization of demanding movement-selection tasks, whether they be oral or manual, than does the temporal lobe. In fact, if we examine in detail the scores of parietal-lobe aphasics on multiple oral movements, they typically get one of the three movements correct on each trial, suggesting that this is the limit of their selection capacity, consistent with their good performance of single oral movements. (In some individuals, we have reason to believe that the parietal function may be subserved by other anterior regions. See Chapter 10 on sex differences.)

The differences between parietal and temporal function are consistent with the different neuroanatomic connections of these two regions, as determined in monkeys. The parietal lobe has significant projections to area 6 (the premotor cortex) and to the basal ganglia, both important for movement control, which the temporal lobe does not have (see Kolb & Whishaw, 1990, for review). In contrast, the temporal lobe receives major input from the auditory cortex and projects to medial temporal regions important in memory function.

Tripartite system

The data suggest that at least two levels of control exist in the left hemisphere for both speech and nonspeech oral movements. One level (anterior) mediates the production of single oral movements in close parallel with single speech sounds. The second level (usually posteriorly based), is necessary for organization of these "single" units into multisyllabic speech, but at this second level there is some divergence of speech and nonspeech movements. Thus the second level may also comprise at least two systems, one of which, based in the temporal lobe, permits selection of speech movements via an auditory-verbal access route. The other, apparently more dependent on the parietal lobe, selects movements without reference to their verbal or nonverbal nature. See Figure 5.1 for a schematic representation of these three systems and their possible interconnections.

It will be recalled that left anterior lesions result in difficulties in reproducing either a single oral movement or a single speech sound. Reproduction of multiple oral movements is also limited by the deficit in reproducing single movements, but this limitation does not hold for certain multisyllabic speech tasks. Where demands on articulation are high, as in rapid changing-syllable repetition ("ba-da-ga"), left anterior damage does indeed cause difficulties, as it does for reproducing several oral movements in a row. However, where the speech to be repeated is in word units and it must simply be repeated at leisure after an auditory presentation, performance in the presence of anterior damage is quite

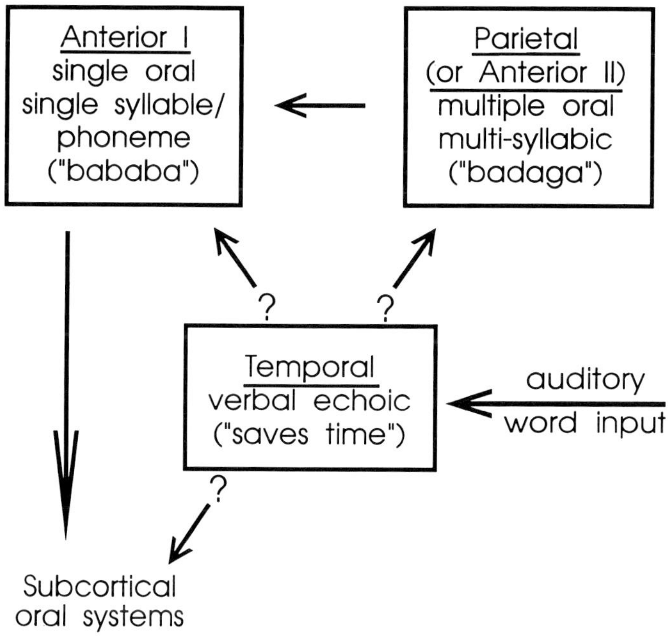

Fig. 5.1 Schema for control of oral/speech movements.

good. Somehow the defective single-syllable system is bypassed, and this appears be mediated by the intact temporal-lobe system, damage to which yields the most severe simple repetition difficulty. Exactly which pathways operate from the temporal lobe in auditory-word repetition is unclear, as the question marks in the figure indicate. Most probably there are alternate routes, depending on availability.

The parietal region, by contrast, is critical for accurate production of several oral movements in a row, and this function extends to speech, insofar as changing-syllable repetition ("ba-da-ga") is affected. However, again with multisyllabic *word* material, damage here has relatively little effect. Thus, although vocal aphasias can for most purposes be usefully regarded as failures of motor programming of the oral musculatures, we must qualify this statement somewhat with respect to *auditory*-verbal control. When basic oral motor selection mechanisms are defective, as they appear to be in certain frontal and parietal lesions on the left, the acoustic-motor pathway vested in the temporal lobe is still able to *reproduce*, though not necessarily *spontaneously produce*, multisyllabic speech. This indicates that when the temporal-lobe echolalic system is intact, it can bypass at least one of the motor programming systems in frontal and parietal regions. Whether it can bypass both systems we do not know, since the answer to this would require fairly extensive damage to both anterior and parietal systems with no invasion of the temporal lobe, an unlikely occurrence in the same patient.

When speech must be self-generated, in contrast, bypassing of neither oral-motor programming system may be possible. In spontaneous speech such as naming, counting, saying days of the week, or describing a picture, there are significant deficits in all aphasic subgroups. Thus all three systems must be intact for completely normal speech function. In self-directed speech (unlike repetition), where syllables must be organized by the speaker into words and phrases, a defect in ability to produce single syllables does limit production of multisyllabic utterances. Hence left anterior pathology is associated with poor fluency, just as inability to reproduce a single oral movement is associated with poor performance of multiple oral movements.

Summary

Repetition of single syllables and reproduction of single oral movements are highly correlated and critically dependent on the left anterior region. Left posterior systems apparently play a very minor role in controlling either speech or nonspeech oral movements of this kind. However, the posterior region does take part in selecting oral movements when more than one must be produced. Within the posterior region, temporal and parietal systems make somewhat different contributions. The parietal lobe in many persons is critical for the selection of articulatory/motor acts whether these involve speech or not. Thus damage to this system results in deficits on multiple oral movements, and on tasks demanding perpetual selection of speech sounds, but has a relatively minor effect on repetition of word-level units. The temporal lobe, however, appears to be critical for selection of speech at a word (rather than an articulatory) level and when damaged results in poor repetition of multisyllabic words or phrases.

Note

1. I thank Dr. R. Teasdell, Department of Rehabilitation Medicine, University Hospital, for providing access to this patient.

6. Manual praxis

One of the most common consequences of pathology to the left cerebral hemisphere has ostensibly nothing to do with communication in the usual sense. This is a symptom called *manual apraxia*, which refers to difficulty in carrying out movements with the hands and arms, not due to weakness or immobility. Historically, manual apraxia was uncovered and is still often assessed by asking patients to show how they would use certain objects, or to demonstrate other "expressive" movements such as waving goodbye to someone, or saluting. The failure to do these things was originally interpreted as a difficulty in making representational movements. A key reason for this interpretation was that manual apraxia was usually found in association with speech disorders, which were a priori viewed as problems in representational function. This view of manual apraxia persisted until fairly recently, and indeed is still held by some, despite the very cogent counterarguments propounded as early as the turn of the century by Hugo Liepmann (1908). Liepmann held very advanced views of both aphasia and apraxia for his time (and even for ours). He suggested that aphasia and apraxia were essentially similar, and that both were manifestations of the loss of an ability to make certain kinds of movements.

Many people who have not seen an aphasic patient nevertheless have no difficulty in accepting the concept of aphasia. Perhaps this is because it is easy to imagine a disturbance of speech, or because we all know, indirectly at least, of people who have suffered from aphasia and it has thus become part of the folklore. But an apraxia is quite unfamiliar, and more difficult for most people to comprehend. Moreover, while a disorder of speech is socially salient and is discovered as soon as one tries to converse with a patient, an apraxia, unless severe, may go undetected in a brief interview. The first time or two that one uncovers an apraxia in a patient, one is impressed by how fundamental and pervasive an intellectual deficit it is.

Apraxia is defined as an inability to carry out specified movements, despite good strength and motility in the muscles or limbs which are affected. Obviously, in assessing this function, we need to be certain that the patient understands what is required. This is particularly important since most apraxic patients are also aphasic, and the apraxia is commonly inferred from a failure to make the required movements to a verbal command. Liepmann (1908) made some excellent suggestions for evaluating the degree to which the apraxia is an artifact of aphasia. If a patient has difficulty only in understanding the *words* "Show me how you salute," s/he would be expected either to look puzzled and do nothing, or to make an inappropriate response but make it accurately. What an apraxic patient does, in contrast, is to either make unrecognizable amorphous movements, or a distorted, crude, or incomplete version of the movement being requested. So instead of saluting, the hand might be brought to the head, but in a totally inappropriate posture and orientation.

Liepmann also proposed a more direct way of ruling out speech comprehension as the basis for the difficulty in making movements. This was to have the patient imitate the movement. Even when the examiner makes the movement first, an apraxic patient typically, although s/he may improve slightly, still has significant difficulty in copying the movement. This failure to produce the movement correctly even with demonstration suggests that apraxia cannot generally be due to simple loss of memory for the movement. Instead, apraxia must involve significant difficulty in making the appropriate postural choices, even when the overall plan or schema is visually presented. Paradoxically, Liepmann (1908, p. 50) often described apraxia as a difficulty in making "movements from memory without guidance from objects." Possibly this conclusion about memory came from the fact that he (and other neurologists) always employed for examination only familiar movements already in the patient's movement repertoire; an inability to generate them might then appear as a failure of retrieval or recall.

Characteristics of manual apraxia

To determine whether the defect in apraxia was in fact limited to familiar movements, Kimura and Archibald (1974) presented a series of meaningless unfamiliar hand and arm movements for immediate reproduction by patients with left- or right-hemisphere damage. The movements, employing a variety of hand postures, arm positions and orientations with respect to the body, bore no resemblance to known gestures or other learned movements. There was an unequivocal deficit in the group of patients with left-hemisphere lesions, compared to those with right-hemisphere lesions (Table 6.1). Data were also available for a small group of age-matched normal persons. In fact, these unfamiliar movements were, if anything, more sensitive to left-hemisphere pathology than were the more traditional tests for apraxia, the "Show me how" kinds of tests. Presumably this is because the unfamiliar movements are simply more difficult for anyone to copy, and moreover were scored in detail, while movements to verbal command are usually scored in a dichotomous pass/fail manner.

Performance on the familiar and unfamiliar kinds of movements was,

Table 6.1 Scores on Movement Copying task, ipsilateral hand

Site of lesion	*N*	Mean/24 (SD)	*p*
Left hemisphere	265	14.9 (6.2)	
Right hemisphere	175	18.9 (3.4)	<.001
Left anterior	29	14.4 (6.2)	
Right anterior	21	18.9 (2.3)	<.001
Left central	23	18.5 (3.8)	
Right central	20	20.1 (3.5)	n.s.
Left posterior	70	15.9 (6.0)	
Right posterior	35	18.7 (3.9)	<.01
Normal controls (first hand)	18	18.8 (3.2)	

however, highly correlated (Pearson $r = .78$), indicating that a single mechanism accounts for much of the movement selection in both. This correlation might have been considerably higher had the tests of praxis to verbal command been as sensitively scored as was the movement copying task. It is also probable that tests of praxis employing verbal commands are likely to be less pure measures of the praxic component, since the element of verbal comprehension may obscure the apraxia. For that reason, *apraxia has been defined in our research sample as a difficulty in copying the unfamiliar movements* described above.

The fact that left-hemisphere lesions had at least as marked an effect on the copying of unfamiliar meaningless movements as on the production or copying of familiar well-practised movements suggests very strongly that the left-hemisphere praxis system is not organized to control only "representational" movements, since the unfamiliar movements do not represent anything else. Nor is it organized only for already learned motor skills. Rather, it appears to be essential for selecting most types of movements or postures of the hands and arms. Naturally, such a system would also be necessary for the learning of motor skills, but its control would not be limited to learned skills. It is important to emphasize this point, because most neurologists and neuropsychologists still persist in interpreting apraxia as a difficulty in organizing *meaningful* movements. It is part of the legacy which has depicted the left hemisphere as specialized for symbolic function, a position we question repeatedly throughout this book.

Motor systems in praxic control

Before we discuss further the nature of manual apraxia, a brief outline of the pertinent motor systems may be useful. There are both crossed and uncrossed connections from the motor cortex to the motor units in the spinal cord. The direct crossed pathways, those without a synapse from cortex to motoneuron in the spinal cord, cross over primarily in what is known as the pyramidal tract (see Fig. 6.1). It is critical for individual movements of the fingers, and is found only in animals which are capable of separate finger movements, primarily primates. Other pathways originating from the cortex are involved in control of more proximal and axial musculature (e.g., shoulders and trunk), and these control systems tend to be more bilateral (Brinkman & Kuypers, 1973).

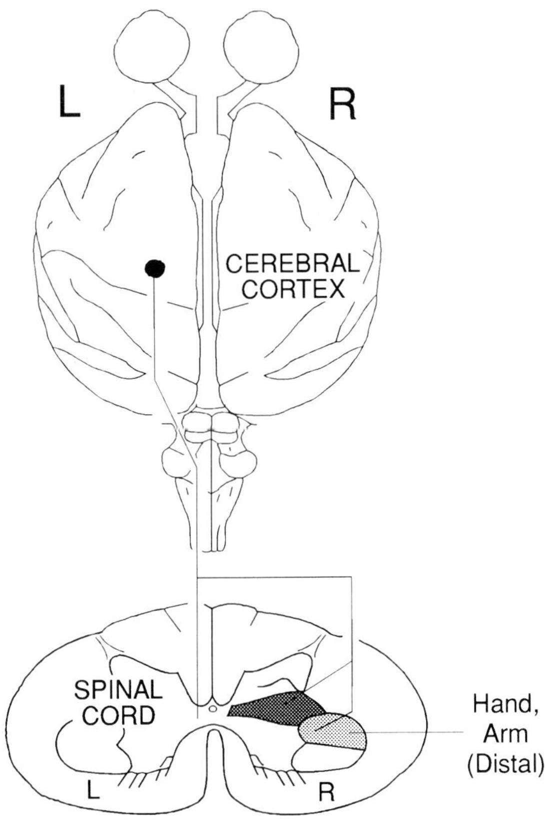

Fig. 6.1 A depiction of the direct corticospinal tract. (After Brinkman & Kuypers, 1973.) Reproduced by permission of the American Association for the Advancement of Science.

Table 6.2 Scores on Movement Copying task in patients with restricted lesions, ipsilateral hand

Site of lesion	*N*	Mean/24 (SD)	*p*
Left anterior	29	14.4 (6.2)	
Right anterior	21	18.9 (2.3)	<.001
Left temporal	26	19.1 (4.8)	
Right temporal	8	20.8 (1.8)	n.s.
Left parietal	14	11.9 (6.1)	
Right parietal	6	16.5 (4.3)	<.10

Additional limb control regions in the cortex are the premotor area, or Brodmann's area 6, and the posterior parietal region, behind the somatosensory cortex. In the monkey, area 6 sends projections to the motor cortex, as well as to brainstem systems which project to regions in the spinal cord controlling primarily proximal and axial muscles. It also receives input from the parietal cortex. Both the premotor and parietal region in monkeys appear to have some function in integrating motor sequences (see Ghez, 1985, for review).

Anterior vs. posterior systems

We saw in Table 6.1 that manual praxis depends on either or both the anterior and posterior regions of the brain in the left hemisphere. Within the group with posterior damage, there were some cases with pathology restricted primarily to the temporal or parietal lobes. These groups are shown in Table 6.2, along with the data from anterior lesions, identical to those in Table 6.1. Only a small number of right-sided cases with temporal or parietal lesions were given this task. However, it is fairly clear that left parietal damage has overall the most severe effect on copying hand movements, followed by left anterior damage. Left temporal damage appears to cause no decrement. The important contribution of the parietal region to hand movement control is not unexpected, in view of its role in such movements in the monkey. We shall see, however, in Chapter 10 on sex differences, that there is marked variation across individuals, in the relative importance of the anterior and parietal regions.

Relation between praxis and corticospinal systems

An assumption often made about the praxis system for which there is little evidence is that its control system is intrinsically bound up with the pyramidal tract (as contrasted with merely operating through this tract). One reason given for this conclusion is that manually apraxic patients have been reported not to have difficulty in making movements of the trunk or other axial musculature, which are known to be independent of the pyramidal system (Geschwind, 1975). However, in a systematic study of apraxic patients, Poeck, Lehmkuhl, and Willmes (1982) convincingly refute the claim that axial movements are unaffected. While it is true that a limb must be mobile in order to make praxic movements, i.e., that the praxis system can probably only operate via an intact corticospinal system, there does not appear to be any relationship between the distribution or control characteristics of the two systems. Some reasons for thinking they are separable are:

1. Apraxia, when it occurs, is typically bilateral, indicating a bilateral praxic control system from the left hemisphere, whereas corticospinal systems are predominantly crossed systems. Thus, patients with manual apraxia from a left-hemisphere lesion may have varying degrees of weakness limited to the right limb, but the apraxic defect will be apparent in the left limb as well.
2. The corticospinal motor systems are particularly essential for distal movement, i.e., for movements of the fingers and hand, while apraxic errors occur in all types of arm movement, including shoulder movement.
3. A mild hemiparesis is not a serious obstacle to copying any movements which do not require fine finger control, suggesting that the praxic programming system is limited by, but not synonymous with, corticospinal systems (Ethelberg, 1951).
4. Related to (3) is the fact that damage restricted to the left Rolandic region and thus extensively involving the corticospinal system does not result in manual apraxia (Tables 6.1 and 6.4).
5. A severe manual apraxia can be, and often is, present without any trace of weakness in the affected limb. This is rather obviously the case in the ipsilateral limb, but may also be true for the right, or contralateral limb as well.
6. To the extent that right-hand preference is a reflection of left-hemisphere praxic function, comparison of left- and right-hand skills does not easily fit a model of greater right preference for the more distal musculature of the arm.

Let us consider first the evidence that apraxia is typically bilateral.

Table 6.3 Relationship of hand strength and tapping speed to manual apraxia

			Strength (kg)				Finger taps (10 sec)			
Lesion group	*N*	Age	Left	(SD)	Right	(SD)	Left	(SD)	Right	(SD)
Left apraxic	29	58.9	28.7	(10.5)	26.8	(10.3)	40.7	(8.7)	38.5	(9.3)
Left nonapraxic	120	46.0	30.95	(10.4)	30.9	(11.7)	42.7	(7.9)	41.5	(10.1)
Right hemisphere	114	46.3	31.1	(9.6)	36.7	(9.7)	36.9	(9.7)	44.8	(8.7)

Most of Liepmann's early cases had significant right hemiparesis, as indeed many cases of left-hemisphere damage with apraxia have today. In such cases, apraxia is only testable in the left arm. The idea unfortunately arose from this that apraxia was a phenomenon especially likely to occur in the left arm, and that it represented primarily a callosal disconnection problem (Geschwind, 1965, 1975). The left arm was presumed to be cut off from the control system in the left hemisphere through a lesion which interrupted pathways crossing between the hemispheres. In the experience of this author, unilateral apraxia is extremely rare in those patients in whom both arms can be tested, i.e., in patients without hemiparesis. If one is careful to screen for adequate strength in the limb, then the scores for copying movements on the two arms are usually quite comparable. (Pearson product–movement correlations between the arms for movement copying scores have always been over .85 in our patient groups.) To illustrate, a review of our patient sample uncovered 50 patients with left-hemisphere lesions who were judged apraxic by their score on copying the unfamiliar movements (less than 13 out of 24), *and* who could be meaningfully tested on both arms. Only 2 of the 50 had a discrepancy of more than 3 points (out of a maximum of 24) between arms. In both these cases, the right arm had the higher score, and had been tested second, presumably benefiting from practise, since identical movements were presented for each arm. It seems reasonable to conclude that these two cases represent random variation, either in performance or in scoring. In neither case was there any more evidence of damage to the commissural systems than in the other cases of left-hemisphere stroke.

The precise pathway(s) by which the left hemisphere exercises control over both limbs are still a matter for speculation. Liepmann's suggestion was that the supramarginal gyrus on the left was the critical center for praxic control. Its access to the motor cortex was assumed to be via the premotor cortex, a suggestion compatible with known pathways from the posterior parietal lobule in the monkey. The premotor area on the left in turn projected to (a) the Rolandic region on the left, which controls the movement of the right hand, and (b) the premotor area in the right hemisphere via the corpus callosum, and thus to the left. With this schema, which is widely accepted, the control of the left hand depends fairly directly on the premotor area of the left hemisphere.

An immediate difficulty with this anatomic schema is that there are no reports of a left-hand apraxia from a right premotor area lesion. The incidence of manual apraxia from a right-hemisphere lesion in right-handers is very low. In our population it is approximately 5% (8 out of 157 right-damaged patients). If we look in detail at the extent of pathology in these 8 cases, 4 of the 8 in fact have restricted *posterior* pathology, and the rest have hemisphere-wide damage. None have pathology restricted to premotor area, nor even to the right anterior region.

In support of the callosal contribution, however, Zaidel and Sperry (1977) report that section of the corpus callosum may result in an impairment in carrying out praxic movements, in the left arm. Their split-brain patients seemed to have their greatest difficulty with movements to verbal command, however, rather than to imitation, indicating that perhaps the difficulty was in transmission of complex verbal messages, rather than in motor control per se. In contrast, Milner and Kolb (1985), using variants of our nonverbal Movement Copying task, report that commissurotomized patients were impaired on *both* hands, relative to patients with focal brain lesions. This would not be predicted from any schema, and if valid (i.e., not an artifact of a short-term memory disorder), would suggest that the corpus callosum carries important crossover fibers from left hemisphere to right hand. These would obviously not be pyramidal fibers. There may, in fact, be alternative routes to bilateral control from the left hemisphere, and one of these may be via the basal ganglia. The fact that really severe apraxias are typically transient argues for such alternatives.

That the left-hemisphere based praxis system is not more critical for distal than proximal movements of the limbs is suggested by the fact that left lesions clearly impair those elements requiring shoulder and elbow movements, as well as postures of the hands. Moreover, simple finger flexion, whether of one or more fingers, was reported by Kimura and Archibald (1974) not to be more affected by left lesions than by right; if anything, the reverse obtained. This conflicts with Geschwind's claim (1975, p. 193) that apraxia is more likely to be manifested in "separate finger movements." When normal persons are asked to flex a finger to a right angle, without moving other fingers, they do this better with the left hand than the right, which also suggests that this is not a function dependent primarily on the left hemisphere (Kimura & Vanderwolf, 1970). Another study on tapping speed in normal subjects by Kimura and Davidson (1975) yielded no systematic change in right-sided preference along the distal–proximal dimension. Thus the shoulder showed as large a percent difference between left and right sides as did the index finger, which is usually employed in studies of tapping speed.

Neither is manual apraxia closely related to the presence of classic pyramidal functions like strength and especially simple repetitive tapping speed. This can be seen in Table 6.3, which shows these basic motor abilities in patients classified as apraxic or not apraxic on the basis of their ability to copy the meaningless movements previously referred to. Normal right-handed subjects generally show about a 4% difference between hands, in favor of the right hand. Assuming that the ipsilateral hand in our patients is approximately normal for these ages, it is apparent that the right hand is affected in the left-hemisphere group, and the left hand is depressed in the right-hemisphere group. Note that patients who are hemiplegic are not included in this table, the data being presented only for patients who could be meaningfully tested on both hands.

Although the apraxic group as a whole has slightly reduced strength and tapping speed in each hand but especially the right, this impairment is small and is probably best accounted for by the older age of the group, since speed and strength both decline with age. The difference between apraxic and nonapraxic left-hemisphere-damaged patients on the left hand is minimal (in contrast to Heilman, 1975), suggesting that simple repetitive finger tapping is not especially sensitive to apraxia. This slight decrement in strength and tapping speed could not in any case *account* for the apraxia, since the most impaired hand on tapping is the left hand of patients with right-hemisphere lesions; yet these individuals do not show apraxia on either hand.

If the corticospinal system in the left hemisphere were a *component*, rather than an end-point, of the praxis system, we would expect that a measure of the strength of the right hand would be a good predictor of apraxia in either hand. Certainly it should be a better predictor than the same measure in the left hand. We can test this very simply by assessing the correlation between left- or right-hand strength, and the score on copying movements, the latter being best taken for the ipsilateral, left, hand. The actual correlation between left-hand movement copying and right-hand strength is .313, which is significant with this large sample (df = 220, $p = <.01$), but accounts for less than 10% of the variance. More pertinent is the fact that the correlation of left-hand movement copying with *left* strength is .231, which is also statistically significant, and the two correlations do not differ significantly. This

Table 6.4 Hand strength, tapping speed, and apraxia in localized lesions

Lesion group	N	Age	Strength (kg)				Finger taps (10 sec)				% Apraxic (score < 13)
			Left	(SD)	Right	(SD)	Left	(SD)	Right	(SD)	
Left anterior	20	51.7	30.4	(9.5)	31.3	(10.5)	43.4	(8.3)	43.6	(10.6)	25%
Right anterior	18	49.2	24.4	(10.4)	30.8	(8.0)	32.8	(9.7)	42.2	(8.9)	0%
Left central	13	41.5	30.7	(10.9)	27.8	(14.5)	44.9	(12.0)	38.3	(9.8)	0%
Right central	15	45.5	26.5	(11.6)	33.2	(11.6)	33.8	(8.0)	43.4	(5.4)	0%
Left posterior	58	42.4	31.4	(10.4)	32.1	(11.2)	42.6	(7.0)	43.7	(8.2)	24%
Right posterior	28	37.7	27.6	(9.0)	31.5	(9.6)	41.2	(8.5)	46.4	(8.7)	4%

indicates quite clearly that right-hand strength in non-hemiplegics is no better an index of apraxia than is left-hand strength. Moreover, analogous correlations in patients with right-hemisphere lesions are of equivalent size, indicating that, unlike apraxia, the effect of weakness is not hemisphere specific.

Even when the cortical component of the corticospinal system is known to be significantly invaded, as in left Rolandic lesions, there is no apraxia present. Liepmann stated quite clearly that damage restricted to the motor cortex, a major component of the corticospinal or pyramidal tracts, would not result in apraxia. In agreement with Liepmann, Table 6.4 shows, in patients with restricted lesions of the hemisphere, that although the patients with left central damage show a moderate right hemiparesis on strength and tapping, none is manually apraxic. (Again, patients who are outright hemiplegic are not included.) The right-hand weakness and slowing is significant, in contrast to that of patients with damage restricted to left anterior or left posterior regions, yet the latter groups show a higher incidence of manual apraxia. The other side of this coin is that many patients with left posterior lesions, who have severe apraxia, have no significant right-hand weakness or slowness, suggesting that the corticospinal system is essentially unaffected. This again indicates that the pyramidal tract plays no special role in praxic control.

Methods of assessment

Much has been made of the fact that many apraxic patients who have difficulty in demonstrating how to use an object in its absence, can nevertheless use the actual object correctly, when it is present. A patient may have difficulty showing how to use a toothbrush, for example, even when the movements are demonstrated, but if given a toothbrush the patient may be much better at making the appropriate movements with it. This is especially likely to be the case if the patient is using the toothbrush as part of a daily routine, as in the context of the bathroom, after breakfast, in familiar surroundings, and so on. The apparent dissociation of object-use demonstration, depending on the presence or absence of the real object, has been particularly emphasized by those who view apraxia, not as a disruption of a functional system, but as a disconnection of one functional system from another.

Geschwind (1967) in particular propounded the latter view, and originally defined apraxia, as "not complex motor," but an "associative disturbance". From this viewpoint, the movement sequence (in hammering a nail, for example) was not in itself disrupted. It was simply not triggered because some necessary pathway to the motor representation was cut off. It was therefore necessary to show that "a movement not made under one set of conditions can be performed in other conditions," hence the emphasis on good object manipulation even when object use could not be demonstrated in the abstract.

There are at least two factors that enter into this observation. One is that there probably often is a significant defect in the use of the actual object, but it is not detected because the movement is not measured finely enough. Another major factor is that with the object present, there are many other cues to assist in selecting the correct movements, i.e., visual, tactual, and possibly kinesthetic. Liepmann (1908) referred to these as "the great crutch which seeing and touching of objects provides—in many cases the hand is led right through the objects, as with scissors—." It appears that the praxic selection mechanism is dispensable, to the extent that other cues are available to aid in selection of the movements. This is different from a disconnection explanation in that the latter implies on all-or-none evocation of the movement pattern.

It therefore seems reasonable, in agreement with Liepmann, to suggest that some apparent *types* of apraxic difficulty are largely reducible to *degrees* of severity, to which different methods of testing were differentially sensitive. A possible scale of difficulty is given below. This crude scaling is for the most part not derived from systematic comparisons within the same patient group. Rather it is extrapolated from piecemeal comparisons and unsystematic compilations in the literature.

1. In the most severe apraxia, there may be difficulty in performing all movements, even everyday well-practised acts in their familiar contexts. Such cases would have difficulty in everyday self-care and eating. Typically, this degree of severity is transient.

2. In less severe apraxia, the grasping of the object to be used may substantially improve performance. Thus a patient may have a hard time going through the motions of certain actions, but insofar as they involve the use of objects, performs substantially better when actually holding the object.

3. Imitating a transitive movement in the absence of an object, or imitating an intransitive movement is generally considered to be more demanding than the above methods of testing for apraxia, and thus likely to show a deficit even when a real object can be used appropriately. Thus, requiring the patient to make the same familiar movement as the demonstrator would uncover such a problem.

4. Demonstrating object use or intransitive movements without prior demonstration and without an object is considered by some to be the most demanding of all the methods generally in use, and thus to be the method most sensitive, and most likely to be disturbed even in mild forms of apraxia. This is the usual method of testing for apraxia in

neurological settings, e.g., "Show me how you use a hammer." It has the disadvantage of being confounded with verbal comprehension problems.

5. Imitating unfamiliar or meaningless movements. Although this is a method not formerly in use, we have found it to be more generally sensitive to a movement disorder than any other task. It has the further advantage that it cannot be confounded wtih aphasic problems. Others have subsequently used this method (deRenzi, Faglioni, & Sorgato, 1982) but without indicating the relative difficulty of the familiar and unfamiliar movements.

On the whole, this appears to be a fairly valid scale, with the possible exception of the ordering of (3) and (4) above. The relative difficulty of these two methods will depend very much on the objects being used, or the movements being required, since not all common object uses or intransitive gestures will be equally frequent or of equivalent difficulty.

The nature of praxic control mechanisms

What can we say about the nature of praxic control mechanisms? Kimura and Archibald (1974), reported that reproduction of single hand postures was much less affected than reproduction of the series of hand movements which comprised the Movement Copying task proper. This remains true in our much larger sample, i.e., the mean score on single Hand Postures of 269 patients with left-hemisphere pathology is 6.8 (SD = 2.6) out of 10, not significantly different from the patients with right-hemisphere pathology ($N = 183$, mean = 7.2, SD = 2.2). However, over time it became clear that left-damaged patients who are apraxic on Movement Copying tend to be impaired in copying single hand postures, their score being 4.8 ($N = 94$, SD = 2.4). The interpretation which seems to best fit these data is that manual apraxia represents a problem in selection of movements such that incorrect movements or postures are frequently chosen instead of the appropriate or correct ones in a situation. When several movements must be selected, as in a series, this puts especially heavy demands on this system, but the difficulty may be detected even when only one movement is required.

If the defective mechanism in apraxia is indeed primarily a selection and not an execution mechanism, then once the movement/posture has been selected, i.e., performed correctly once, repeating it should not present further difficulty. This does appear to be the case, in that manual tasks which require simply the repetition of the same (single) movement, are not affected by left-hemisphere damage any more than by right; whereas motor tasks in which constant changes in hand/arm posture are required, prove difficult for patients with left damage.

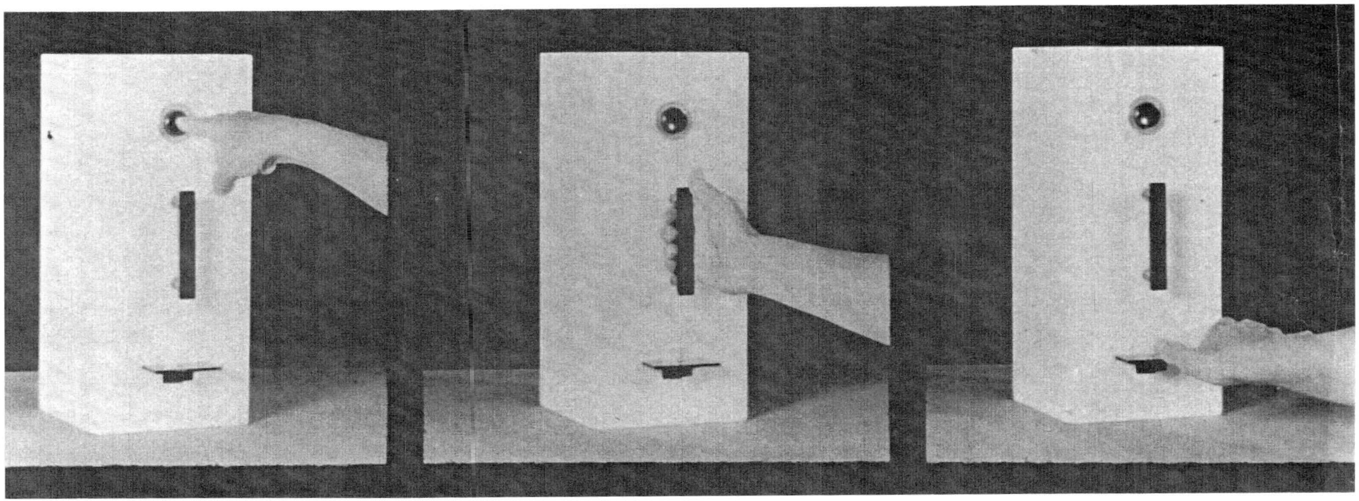

Fig. 6.2 The Manual Sequence Box (Kimura, 1977).

This difference is well illustrated by comparing two tasks. The first, the Manual Sequence Box task, shown in Fig. 6.2, requires the subject to learn a simple series of hand movements—press the top button with the index finger, pull forward on the vertical bar with all four fingers, and press down on the bottom horizontal bar with the lateral side of the thumb. Normal persons learn this, after a demonstration, to a criterion of five successive correct trials in less than half a minute. However, many patients with left-hemisphere pathology cannot learn the task even after several minutes of trying, and with repeated immediate feedback, and further demonstration (Kimura, 1977). Those who do learn it to criterion take much longer than patients with right-hemisphere damage. This slowness of acquisition is again apparent no matter which hand acquires the task.

Some, severely apraxic patients, never approximate the correct movements. Most patients, however, do acquire the three movements, mixed in with other irrelevant ones, but they do not emit them at the appropriate places on the box. It is worth pointing out that apraxic patients do not typically confuse the spatial direction of the external array itself, that is, they go from top to bottom, just like everyone else. The most common error is a perseverative error, the repetition of a movement just completed. Thus, if the thumb has just been used on the bottom bar, the patient will often continue with the thumb to the buzzer at the top of the box, rather than using the index finger, which is the correct response. Indeed, some of the increased time to acquire the task in those who do so could be seen to involve a correction process. Patients often corrected themselves from an initially wrong (and often perseveratory) posture. Performance on the Manual Sequence Box task suggested a number of things. Most important perhaps was that the defect in left-hemisphere apraxia was not simply an ordering or sequencing defect. Patients who were impaired were not merely making appropriate hand and arm postures at the wrong place or in the wrong order. Rather, they were often making completely incorrect movements. The strong tendency to perseverate suggested that changing from one posture to another was very difficult in the presence of apraxia. Perhaps, if one has a defective selection mechanism, the most available movement is the one just completed. This indicates that simply repeating a movement over and over should be a relatively easy task.

The next task—the Nut-and-Bolt task—employs such repetition, and again requires manipulation of an object by the hand. The subject is required to turn a nut up and down a bolt (Fig. 6.3), using fingers and thumb. S/he is allowed first to practise the movement a couple of times before each traversal, to ensure that the instructions are understood. The score is the average time taken to complete the up and the down trial, for each hand separately. Data on this task contrast sharply with

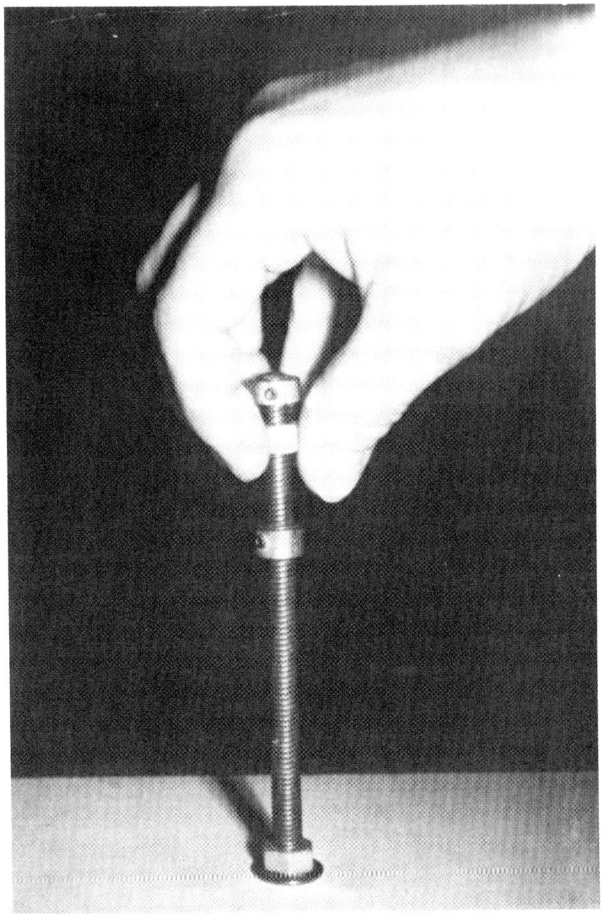

Fig. 6.3 The Nut-and-Bolt task (Kimura, 1979).

those on the Box task. On the Nut-and-Bolt task, patients with left-hemisphere damage have no special difficulty, compared to patients with right-hemisphere damage. These findings are entirely consistent with those of Pieczuro and Vignolo (1967), on a task requiring unscrewing of bolts from a board, on which their patients with left- or right-hemisphere lesions did not differ.

As can be seen in Fig. 6.4, the hand ipsilateral to the lesion performs the task in about 10 sec, on average, regardless of the side of the damage, or of the locus within the hemisphere. The hand contralateral to the damage, however, is significantly slower than the ispilateral hand, especially if the anterior/central region is affected by the damage. The

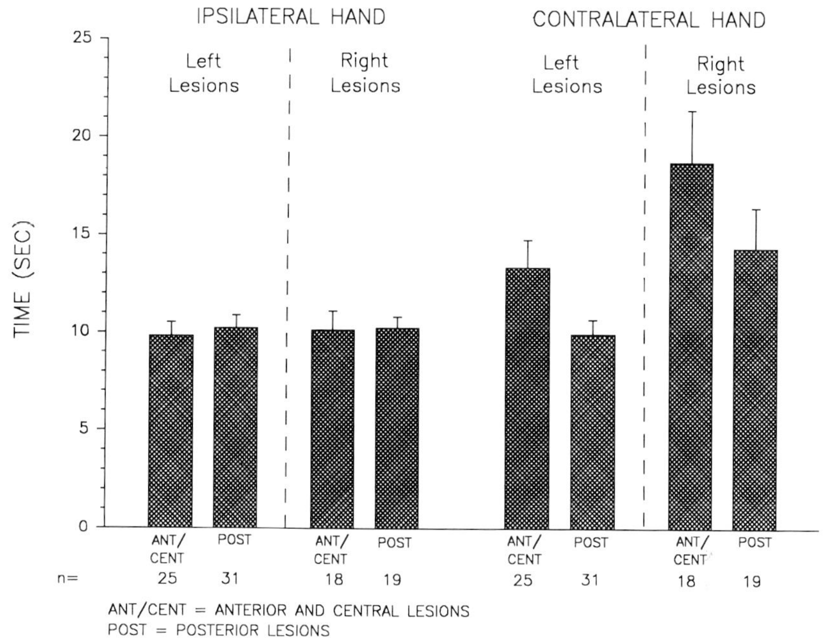

Fig. 6.4 Performance on the Nut-and-Bolt task after ipsilateral and contralateral lesions of the left and right hemispheres.

contralateral deficit is at least as great after right-hemisphere damage as after left. This is precisely what we would expect if only or primarily corticospinal systems were involved in controling these movements.

Recall that on the Box task, and on Movement Copying, scores on both ipsilateral and contralateral hands are affected by appropriate left-hemisphere damage. This means that if we compare performance across various motor tasks for the ipsilateral hand only, we can see the effect of apraxia without the confound of contralateral weakness or clumsiness. Figure 6.5 shows the ipsilateral hand only, for those patients who actually learned the Box task to criterion. Thus we are already excluding patients so apraxic that they could not learn the Box task. Their times are shown for an additional five speeded trials on the Box task, after acquisition, as well as for the Nut-and-Bolt task.

The apraxic patients are not significantly slowed on the Nut and Bolt task, compared to nonapraxic patients, but they are significantly slower on the speeded phase of the Box task. This indicates that the chief reason for their poor performance on the Box is not the learning or memory component (since they have already learned the task and are not making errors now), but rather the fact that they must constantly

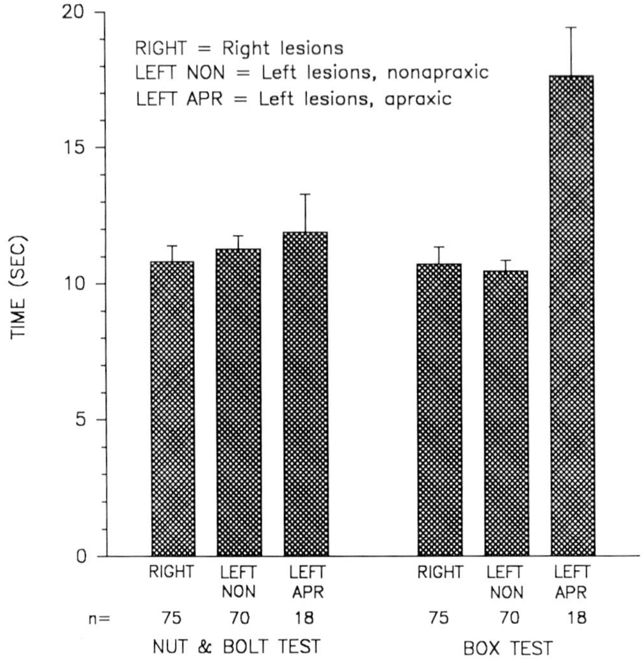

Fig. 6.5 Performance on two disparate motor tasks after left or right lesions (ipsilateral hand).

select new hand movements, which they do not have to do on Nut and Bolt.

Relationship between oral and manual control

There are some obvious parallels between the nature of the oral and manual control systems which depend on the left hemisphere, but there are also some differences. We have just seen that the speeded repetition of a single manual movement, as in repetitive finger-tapping, or the Nut-and-Bolt task, is not selectively affected by left-hemisphere damage relative to right. This contrasts with the speeded repetition of single speech sounds, which *is* selectively affected by left-hemisphere pathology, but is critically dependent on the left anterior system. A similar contrast obtains for simple unspeeded repetition of single oral movements and single hand postures, that is, the oral movements show a left anterior dependence while the hand postures are not significantly affected either by generalized left-hemisphere pathology or by left anterior pathology.

Although patients who are manually apraxic as defined by the Movement Copying task, tend also to be impaired on the single hand postures, it was suggested earlier that these findings reflected the operation of the same system in both cases. The Movement Copying task, requiring several movements, is simply much more sensitive to the selection deficit. This is again unlike oral movement control systems, in that multiple oral movements appear not to make merely additional demands on the anteriorly based single oral system, but to involve a separate area.

This second or multiple-oral movement system, which is often but not necessarily posterior-based (see Chapter 10 on sex differences), appears to share some features with the manual system. We saw in Chapter 5 that the correlation between scores on the Multiple Oral task and the manual Movement Copying task was .67, which suggests significant overlap between the two, though not a tight association. The commonality appears in the programming of movement selection when more than one movement must be executed. Damage to this programming system does not prevent the speeded repetition of single speech or single manual movements ("ba-ba-ba", Nut-and-Bolt tasks), but does impair the speeded repetition of changing movements ("ba-da-ga", Box task). However, since the oral and manual commands ultimately go to different effectors, they necessarily diverge at some point, limiting the functional overlap between the two systems.

Praxis as movement within personal space

The fact that the cues provided by the handling of real objects can generally substitute for a defective praxis system indicates that the system is especially important for selecting movements in the absence of external sensory information; for "movements without objects," as Liepmann put it. This seems to be a system for programming or selecting movements with the body as framework, with minimal external guidance. A rough parallel in motor control theory is the term "open loop," as compared to "closed loop," the latter being a movement modifiable by feedback. Another roughly comparable term is "ballistic" movement, implying that the movement is preprogrammed and will not be alterable by sensory information after its initiation.

In reality, nearly all movements involve both open- and closed-loop control to some degree, in a constant interaction between preprogramming and the modification which depends on external information to reset or redirect the movements. Assuming that much of the programming of our complex arm and hand movements is done by the left hemisphere, and that much of the spatial locating of external stimuli is done by the right hemisphere, then most activities would demand the bihemispheric integration of these two systems to varying degrees. Most sports, especially those involving responses to moving targets, would require such integration to a high degree.

In contrast, a movement like mixing a cake with a whisk, would require minimal external control, once the first movement or two had established the dimensions of the bowl vis-à-vis the whisk. Much of it could be done with the eyes closed, and with only a periodic tactual–kinesthetic reminder of the bowl dimensions. Many of the everyday motor skills we use are of the latter kind, where the external stimuli are immobile or relatively unvarying, e.g., cutting bread, opening doors with a key, switching lights on and off, hammering, and so on. These are all fairly demanding of motor programming, but not of spatial analysis, and would therefore be expected to depend primarily on the left hemisphere for organization.

Perception of movements after left-hemisphere damage

We may ask whether left-hemisphere pathology affects the ability to process or perceive the hand movements presented for reproduction. This obviously could not *account* for the apraxia, since these same patients have difficulty also when required to generate similar movements to verbal command. Moreover, the general expectation from the visual nature of the presentation would be that the right hemisphere would be involved in movement perception to a significant degree. However, it is quite possible that, when presented with arm and hand movements *to be reproduced*, they may be processed with reference to the same left-hemisphere system used to generate them, and thus that perception might be faulty also. This is similar to the suggestion that speech sounds are perceived via a mechanism which overlaps substantially with the neural articulatory system (Liberman, 1982). It would in that case be difficult and probably uninformative to attempt to separate the perceptual from the production components in the case of hand movements to be imitated.

Instead, a task was devised to answer the question whether processing of movements presented in the same space as praxic movements, but requiring no reproduction, would be selectively affected by left-hemisphere damage. The experimenter moved the arms in the same general area in which the Movement Copying task was presented, tracing in the air an unfamiliar symmetrical figure which the patient had to select from a multiple-choice array (Fig. 6.6). This task was given to a consecutive series of 77 left-damaged cases and 59 right-damaged cases.

It is clear from Table 6.5 that left-sided cases show no impairment relative to right, although they are impaired on the Movement Copying task. It appears, therefore, that the processing of limb movement

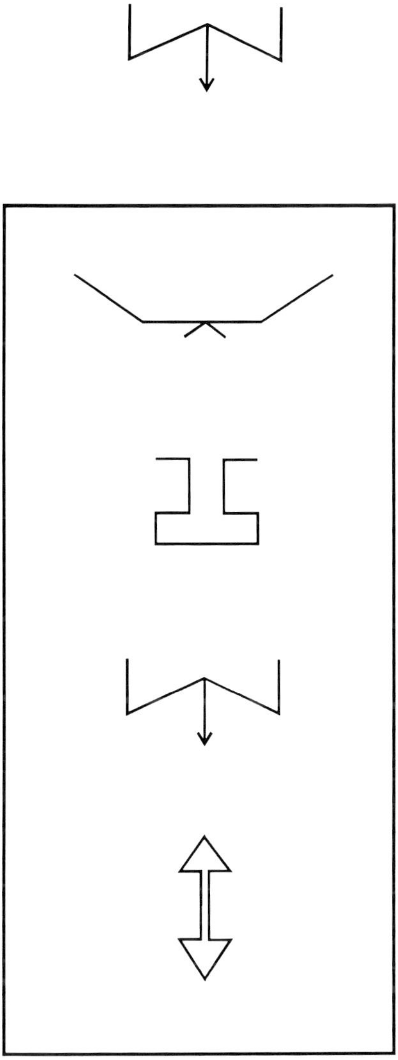

Fig. 6.6 An example of the hand-generated patterns traced for identification by the patient. The top figure is executed by the experimenter, and the patient selects it from a card containing the four figures shown.

Table 6.5 Identification of hand shapes

Side of Lesion	*N*	Copying hand movements/24	Identifying hand shapes/12
Left mean	77	14.5 (60%)	9.0 (75%)
(SD)		(5.7)	(2.1)
Right mean	59	18.8 (78%)	9.2 (77%)
(SD)		(3.7)	(2.6)
p =		<.001	n.s.

per se is no more affected by left damage than by right. This confirms the position that manual apraxia is not a result of a deficit in processing hand movements in visual space.

Types of apraxia

At least two subtypes of apraxia are described in the literature, which may not be reducible to differences in degree or severity. These are ideational apraxia and ideomotor apraxia. The latter is the easier to define and comprehend, in that it refers to the inability to generate a correct movement, whether the movement is stipulated by verbal command or by demonstration for imitation. It thus comprises a basic motor selection defect. Slight discrepancies between performance to command and by imitation are assumed to be related to the ease or difficulty of the respective movements, past frequency of occurrence, and so on. It is ideomotor apraxia which most apraxic patients suffer from, and to which most writers on the subject refer. The Movement Copying task described earlier, which we have used to define apraxia, will of course identify ideomotor apraxia.

Ideational apraxia is more variably defined, but it usually refers to an impairment of the overall plan of a complex series of movements, such as might be involved, for example, in lighting a cigarette. It was inferred to be a separable phenomenon, from the fact that the occasional patient, who could copy components of a movement quite well, could not generate the movements spontaneously to verbal command, without a model of the movement (Liepmann, 1908; Poeck, 1983). We must consider the possibility that so-called ideational apraxia may simply represent a milder version of ideomotor apraxia, in that it manifests itself only in the most demanding situation, the spontaneous generation of a series of movements to command. In fact, Zangwill (1960), in reviewing several cases of presumed ideational apraxia in the literature, found none which did not also have ideomotor apraxia. Thus using the scaling method outlined earlier, it appeared that demonstrating object use from memory (method 4) was only slightly worse than imitation (method 3).

Other reports, however, claim that ideational apraxia as a dissociable syndrome may exist but is very rare. Poeck (1983) suggests that less than 5% of patients with left-hemisphere damage suffer from ideational apraxia, much less than the number who suffer from aphasia or ideomotor apraxia. This small minority of apraxic individuals shows a distinctive pattern of behavioral deficits, i.e., the discrepancy between intact imitation and impaired spontaneous production of specified movements is said to be large and reliable (Liepmann, 1980; Heilman, 1973; Lehmkuhl & Poeck, 1981). These reports also claim that speech comprehension difficulty was effectively ruled out as the basis for the apraxia, though all cases were aphasic. These patients have no particular difficulty in actually handling objects, as is true of the vast majority of patients with either ideomotor or ideational apraxia.

A somewhat anomalous definition of ideational apraxia, in view of the studies cited above, is that it is an inability to correctly handle objects with intact ability to imitate (deRenzi, Pieczuro, & Vignolo, 1968). DeRenzi and coworkers reported that a number of patients, who could not use real objects placed before them in an examination situation, could nevertheless copy quite well some common intransitive gestures. We must assume, although we are not told, that they could also copy the demonstration of object use. Since we have actually very little information about the relative difficulty of some of these methods of assessment, we must be cautious about prematurely inferring dissociations. Other possible interpretations of the claimed dissociation is that there may be a mixture of ideational and ideomotor apraxia present; or, that the relative difficulty of the object-movements and the intransitive gestures chosen was different for different individuals.

Poeck and coworkers hypothesize that the ideational apraxia they describe is a defect superordinate to the components of the movement sequence, such that picking up the match, striking it, and so on, may in themselves be correctly performed, but the overall act is defective (Lehmkuhl & Poeck, 1981; Poeck, 1983). Conceptualizations of this kind lead us to expect that ideational apraxics should make primarily *ordering* errors. Were this so, there would be a strong basis for considering this to be a failure at a different level from ideomotor apraxia. Descriptions of patients with ideational apraxia indicate, however, that this is by no means always the case. Many of the movements generated are of the aimless nondescript kind which are typical of ideomotor apraxia. Poeck also reports perseveration as a frequent response, a characteristic of ideomotor apraxia (Kimura, 1977). However, in support of the idea that ideational apraxia involves a defect of action planning is the finding that, whereas such patients cannot correctly order a series of pictures depicting activities like dialing a telephone, they are comparable to other patients in arranging pictures which do not depict praxic activities (Lehmkuhl & Poeck, 1981). We do not know whether the presence of ideomotor apraxia might not be sufficient to cause such an ordering impairment. Nor do we know that the ideational apraxics can copy unfamiliar movements accurately, although the implication would be that they can. Given all these limitations on the data, and the very low incidence of reports of ideational apraxia, its existence as a separate entity must remain open to question.

Summary

One of the most common consequences of left-hemisphere pathology is manual apraxia, a disturbance in making hand movements, whether elicited by verbal command or by imitation. This difficulty can occur quite independent of motor weakness, and when both arms can be tested, manifests itself bilaterally. It appears to reflect the function of motor programming systems outside the Rolandic region, in frontal and parietal lobes. These praxis systems are especially important for controlling movement within personal space, with the body as framework. There is significant overlap between the manual praxis system and systems responsible for organizing multiple oral movements and speech, described in Chapter 5.

7. Constructional ability

Constructional apraxia refers to an impairment in forming designs, objects, or materials with the hands, under visual guidance. It is also called visuoconstructive disability. The specific activities sampled typically include drawing (with or without a model), making a specified design with blocks (Block Design), assembling pieces to make a coherent picture (Object Assembly), making a design out of sticks, and so on. Although many writers on the subject have emphasized the role of the right hemisphere in visuoconstructive ability, there clearly is a contribution from the left hemisphere as well; and this contribution appears to relate to its role in motor control.

Constructional apraxis, in fact, was originally defined by Kleist in such a way as to focus on left-hemisphere symptomatology, in his words "a disturbance in constructional activity [with] adequate form perception and discrimination and preserved ability to localize objects in visual space" (cited by Benton, 1972). These qualifications were subsequently ignored when it became apparent that many patients with right-hemisphere damage, albeit with visuospatial disturbances, showed deficits in constructional ability which were, superficially at least, quite similar to those with left-hemisphere damage.

Paradoxically, it soon became axiomatic in the neurological literature that constructional deficits were more common after *right*-sided lesions than after left (Paterson & Zangwill, 1944; McFie, Piercy, & Zangwill, 1950). Within the right hemisphere, the right parietal region was claimed to be particularly critical for visuoconstructional ability (Piercy, Hècaen, & Ajuriaguerra, 1960). However, most studies claiming such right-hemisphere predominance did not include left-damaged patients who were aphasic. Although such omissions were sometimes intended to ensure that the patient understood the procedure, the consequence was that the most impaired left-damaged patients were excluded, making any comparison with right-damaged patients problematic (Benton, 1973).

When care is taken not to exclude patients with severe aphasia, the paramount contribution of the right hemisphere to constructional ability has not been confirmed (Colombo, deRenzi, & Faglioni, 1976; Arena & Gainotti, 1978; Kimura & Faust, 1987). We can usually safely infer, in aphasics, that the procedure has been understood if the patient has done a simpler item of the same kind, or if the attempts approximate the correct solution even though not entirely correct.

Table 7.1 Incidence of unrecognizable drawings and of contralateral omissions (house and person combined)

Number of:	Left total	Right total	Left nonparetic	Right nonparetic
Drawings	362	265	279	170
Unrecognizable[a]	40 (11%)	17 (6%)	20 (7%)	4 (2%)
With neglect on drawings[b]	2 (0.5%)	16 (6%)	0	3 (2%)

[a] χ^2 (total groups) = 4.74, df = 1, $p < .04$.
[b] χ^2 (total groups) = 16.51, df = 1, $p = < .01$.

Spontaneous drawing

In our large series of cases with unilateral cerebral pathology, we always attempted to include aphasic patients. Considering first the spontaneous drawings of either a house or person, which we had collected over several years, we found that the number of drawings labeled as unrecognizable to an unbiassed observer was in fact significantly higher in the group of patients with left-hemisphere damage (Table 7.1). A common example of this might be a box-like structure drawn instead of a house. In this sample, severe drawing disability in the left-hemisphere group was associated with aphasia and apraxia, whereas in the right-hemisphere group, it appeared to be associated with extensive damage to the hemisphere, as judged by degree of hemiparesis and incidence of field defects (Kimura & Faust, 1987). A similar suggestion had been made by Arrigoni and deRenzi (1964).

On other measures of drawing ability, equivalent left- and right-damaged groups did show some qualitative differences. Thus, the left-damaged groups produced fewer lines and smaller drawings (but only a trend toward getting fewer details correct); while the right-damaged patients showed a higher degree of rotation on the page, and more neglect in the drawings themselves (Tables 7.1 and 7.2). These findings on qualitative differences between the effects of left and right pathology are compatible with suggestions from earlier studies (Piercy & coworkers, 1960; Warrington, 1969). Such studies also suggested that providing a model improves performance in patients with left-hemisphere damage, but not in right-damaged cases.

No support was found in our data for the presumption that the right parietal region was particularly critical for constructional, including drawing, ability. The most impaired of all was the group with left anterior

Table 7.2 Mean scores on drawings

	Left total (N = 191)		Right total (N = 140)			Left nonparetic (N = 149)		Right nonparetic (N = 90)		
	Mean	(SD)	Mean	(SD)	p	Mean	(SD)	Mean	(SD)	p
House drawing										
Number of details/17	8.2	(2.3)	8.7	(1.8)	.029	8.4	(2.2)	8.9	(1.6)	.059
Distortion ratio (max. = 1.00)	0.58	(0.27)	0.54	(0.23)	.159	0.52	(0.24)	0.48	(0.21)	.223
Number of lines	36.8	(23.8)	43.8	(30.1)	.019*	39.4	(25.2)	44.9	(29.9)	.132
Size (in^2)	13.2	(11.2)	14.1	(11.5)	.483	13.3	(10.9)	14.6	(11.2)	.351
Time per line (sec)	3.2	(2.8)	2.8	(2.7)	.218	3.1	(2.8)	2.3	(1.8)	.036
Time per detail (sec)	12.7	(9.9)	12.95	(13.0)	.906	12.6	(10.2)	10.6	(8.3)	.168
Rotation (degrees)	4.1	(2.9)	5.1	(3.4)	.116	3.7	(2.2)	4.25	(3.0)	.017*
Person drawing										
Number of details/13	9.3	(3.3)	10.1	(3.5)	.053	9.9	(3.2)	10.8	(3.4)	.062
Distortion ratio (max. = 1.00)	0.57	(0.30)	0.50	(0.30)	.057	0.51	(0.29)	0.44	(0.29)	.115
Size (in^2)	11.9	(12.0)	15.7	(12.0)	.009**	12.5	(12.4)	15.7	(12.0)	.070
Time per detail (sec)	12.9	(11.0)	14.1	(19.7)	.570	13.7	(12.0)	11.7	(9.3)	.273

* $p < .02$.
** $p < .01$.

Table 7.3 Mean scores on drawings (localized groups)

	Left anterior (N = 21)		Left parietal + (N = 13)		Right anterior (N = 14)		Right parietal + (N = 16)	
	Mean	(SD)	Mean	(SD)	Mean	(SD)	Mean	(SD)
House drawing								
Number of details/17[a], **	6.7	(2.4)	7.5	(1.9)	8.5	(1.7)	8.4	(1.4)
Distortion ratio*	0.74	(0.26)	0.62	(0.19)	0.59	(0.27)	0.54	(0.20)
Number of lines*	26.8	(12.9)	34.4	(16.9)	45.0	(32.4)	47.9	(46.4)
Size (in^2)	13.0	(13.1)	19.0	(15.0)	18.5	(13.4)	16.2	(14.2)
Time per line (sec)[b], **	3.0	(1.3)	5.9	(6.0)	2.2	(1.1)	1.9	(1.0)
Time per detail (sec)	12.7	(8.3)	19.2	(17.3)	10.8	(8.2)	8.0	(4.6)
Rotation (degrees)	5.6	(2.6)	5.0	(4.7)	5.5	(3.9)	3.3	(1.5)
Person drawing								
Number of details/13*	8.0	(3.1)	8.3	(3.4)	8.7	(2.9)	10.0	(4.5)
Distortion ratio*	0.66	(0.30)	0.61	(0.25)	0.57	(0.28)	0.57	(0.32)
Size (in^2)	11.4	(15.6)	14.1	(13.3)	21.9	(17.1)	15.8	(11.1)
Time per detail (sec)	16.9	(19.3)	16.6	(18.6)	9.5	(6.7)	10.7	(11.2)

* $p < .05$.
** $p < .01$.
[a] Left anterior and right parietal groups differ significantly.
[b] All groups differ significantly from the left parietal group.

Fig. 7.1 Examples of house drawings from two manually apraxic patients with left-hemisphere lesions. The figure on the left was drawn in the upper left corner of the page.

lesions, who produced fewer lines, fewer correct details, more distortion and smaller drawings than any other group (Table 7.3). Several of their house drawings consisted merely of a small rectangle, with minimal details pertaining to a house (Fig. 7.1). Such "oversimplification" has been noted by several previous investigators (Piercy & coworkers, 1960; Arrigoni & deRenzi, 1964; Gainotti & Tiacci, 1970). Patients with left posterior damage which included (but was not restricted to) the parietal region were the slowest of all groups in completing their drawings. They also showed trends for fewer lines, fewer details, and more distortion than other groups, with the exception of left anterior.

WAIS constructional tasks

Similar findings obtain on other constructional tasks. There is no difference in mean score between left- and right-damaged groups on the Block Design and Object Assembly subtests of the Wechsler Adult Intelligence Scale (1955) (Table 7.4). Thus, we find little support for the claim of right-hemisphere dominance on these tasks. Moreover, if we consider only those cases in each group who obtain low scores, i.e., Block Design raw score less than 13, there is again no significant difference between groups in the incidence of such scores (see Table 7.5). The apparently lower score of such patients with right-hemisphere damage is due to the greater number of cases in this group scoring zero. On this measure, the left and right groups do differ significantly. However, one must keep in mind that those scoring zero constitute only about 8% of the patients with right-hemisphere pathology and 3% of patients with left-hemisphere pathology. They are thus not representative of most patients with unilateral brain lesions.

Within this small subgroup of patients who score zero on Block Design, we find that, in the left-damaged group, 8 of the 9 patients are aphasic, 8 out of 9 are apraxic, 5 have significant hemiparesis, and 3

Table 7.4 Means for two constructional tasks

Group	*N*	Age	Performance IQ	Block Design (max. = 48)	Object Assembly (max. = 44)
All left-sided cases	266	50.4	94.8	23.7 (11.3)	23.5 (10.1)
All right-sided cases	167	48.3	92.9	23.1 (12.8)	22.1 (10.0)
Left aphasic	90	57.4	86.2	16.8 (10.8)	18.0 (9.7)
Left nonaphasic	175	46.2	98.4	27.4 (9.5)	26.0 (9.2)
Left apraxic	86	58.2	83.2	14.0 (9.2)	16.0 (9.2)
Left nonapraxic	169	46.8	99.3	28.1 (9.1)	26.7 (8.4)
Right apraxic	9	61.3	76.2	6.9 (9.0)	9.6 (9.6)
Right nonapraxic	145	47.8	94.9	24.6 (12.5)	23.2 (9.6)

Table 7.5 Incidence of low Block Design scores

Cases given test	Below 13 (raw)[a]	Mean scores	Zero scores[b]
Left-sided = 277	57 (20.5%)	7.1 (4.4)	9 (3%)
Right-sided = 192	51 (27%)	4.4 (4.1)	16 (8%)

[a] $\chi^2 = 2.29$ (df = 1, $p < .15$, n.s.).
[b] $\chi^2 = 5.81$ (df = 1, $p < .02$).

have visual field defects; 2 have restricted anterior and 2 have restricted posterior lesions. In the right-hemisphere group, 13 of the 16 have significant hemiparesis, 13 have left field defects, 3 have restricted posterior lesions, and 1 has a restricted anterior lesion. Thus, as for drawing, very poor performance on Block Design appears to be associated with more extensive pathology in the right hemisphere than is true for the left hemisphere.

To consider the effect of locus of lesion in another way, we looked at patients with pathology restricted to anterior, posterior or central sectors of the hemispheres (Table 7.6). Again there are no significant differences in constructional scores between equivalent left and right groups, whether we look at mean scores on Block Design and Object Assembly subtests, or at incidence of low scores. The same is true of more restricted damage within the posterior sector (Table 7.7). Of

Table 7.6 Mean scores on WAIS constructional tests in localized cases

Locus	Age	*N*	Block Design	Object Assembly	Block Design < 13	Patients with score = 0
Left anterior	53.6	28	19.0 (10.9)	20.1 (8.7)	10	2
Right anterior	51.2	24	22.2 (9.6)	24.2 (7.1)	4	1
Left central	41.7	22	31.5 (8.2)	28.4 (8.6)	0	0
Right central	42.2	19	30.8 (8.9)	27.3 (7.1)	1	0
Left posterior	42.8	73	25.9 (11.6)	25.4 (10.1)	11	2
Right posterior	39.8	39	27.8 (13.2)	24.1 (10.0)	4	3

Note: None of the differences between equivalent left–right groups is significant.

Table 7.7 WAIS constructional tests in localized posterior groups

Locus	Age	*N*	Block Design	Object Assembly	Block Design < 13	Patients with score = 0
Left temporal	35.3	29	30.0 (11.2)	28.1 (9.3)	1	0
Right temporal	37.4	10	32.8 (9.2)	26.0 (6.5)	0	0
Left parietal	41.9	9	24.4 (13.8)	28.0 (11.2)	2	1
Right parietal	44.3	6	20.0 (17.2)	17.7 (12.6)	2	2
Left occipital	41.9	14	29.7 (9.4)	27.1 (9.9)	1	0
Right occipital	41.0	5	34.6 (5.0)	28.8 (6.4)	0	0

Note: None of the differences between equivalent left–right groups is significant.

particular interest are the left and right parietal groups. The sample sizes here are small, so that null statements are problematic, but given those limitations, no significant differences emerge. (There is a weak trend for Object Assembly scores to be lower in patients with right parietal lesions.) This at least suggests that no *striking* overall differences exist in the contribution of the left and right parietal regions to constructional ability, and is compatible with our findings for spontaneous drawing. The same may be said with more confidence for temporal and occipital lobes, where the sample sizes are slightly larger, and the differences even more negligible.

However, although there may be no gross difference in final scores between left and right cases, there have been reports that the nature of the constructional deficit is different in the two groups. Largely because there are frequent spatial or perceptual impairments after right-hemisphere pathology, the inference has been made that the constructional disability resulting from right-sided lesions is related more to perceptual and spatial-processing difficulties. It is also anecdotally accepted that patients with right-hemisphere lesions tend more often to produce disorganized arrays of blocks on a block design task, in comparison with left-sided cases. This may be true even in the absence of a gross neglect of space. We have similarly found that, even when left apraxic patients earn low scores on the Block Design test, their block arrays are nearly always in neat squares, albeit with incorrect patterns. Nevertheless, interesting as these clinical observations are, they do not permit unequivocal inferences about the respective contributions of the two hemispheres to constructional ability.

Relation to manual apraxia

Deficits in Copying Movements (see Chapter 6), a measure of manual apraxia, bear a strong relation to deficits in visuoconstructional ability, particularly in patients with left-hemisphere lesions (Kimura, 1986; and see Table 7.4). Thus the correlation between Copying Movements and the raw score on Block Design is .70 for the entire left-hemisphere group (df = 239, $p < .001$). This means that variations in degree of manual apraxia account for about 50% of the variance on the Block Design task. Even in patients with right-hemisphere damage, the correlation is highly significant ($r = .44$, df = 162, $p < .02$). However, the difference between the correlations is also significant ($p < .02$), indicating that the relationship is closer in the left-damaged group, as might be expected. This does not appear to be merely a consequence of a restricted range in the right-damaged group, since their scores on movement copying range from 7 to 24, and only 8 out of 175 cases achieve the maximum score of 24, ruling out a ceiling effect.

Both in spontaneous drawings, and on the WAIS constructional tests (Table 7.4), it is apparent that performance is worst in patients who are manually apraxic. (Although this is most salient in patients with left-hemisphere lesions, since they form the bulk of manually apraxic cases, the small group of right manual apraxics is also severely affected on constructional tasks. None of them is aphasic.) The striking difference between apraxic and non-apraxic patients is compatible with suggestions that the left hemisphere normally contributes an "executive" component to constructional activities (Piercy & coworkers, 1960). Yet no information is available on precisely how the behavior of a left-damaged constructional apraxic is different from that of a right-damaged patient with constructional difficulties. Therefore, in an attempt to analyze the characteristics of the presumed motor contribution, a number of patients with unilateral damage were videotaped doing a variety of constructional tasks. A detailed movement-by-movement

Table 7.8 Movement sample on a three-dimensional eight-block design

Measure	Left group (14)	Left apraxic (6)	Left nonapraxic (8)	Right group (8)
Flip ratio	.01	.01	.01	.03
Rotate ratio	.02	.01	.02	.03
Slide ratio	.05	.06	.04	.02
Pickup ratio	.17	.13	.19	.16
Total events	14.8	14.3	15.5	16.9
Total movements	11.9	14.3	10.0	12.6
Events/time	.33	.24	.40	.33
Movements/event	1.52	1.71	1.45	1.58

analysis was completed on several three-dimensional constructional tasks, one of which is the copy of an eight-block design (Benton, Hamsher, Varney, & Spreen, 1983).

Our observer (R. Faust[1]), after viewing several tapes at random, generated a list of all possible movements which occurred, and subsequently tallied every movement for each patient he viewed. This was done without formal knowledge of the patient's praxic status, but it rapidly becomes apparent to anyone with experience, which patients are having difficulties, so that a "blind" observational situation is not possible. However, we had no specific predictions about what would happen, and there is no reason to think that the tally was affected by any particular hypothesis.

The data in Table 7.8 are shown for the most commonly occurring movements, in a small group of patients with left- or right-damage, and within the left-damaged group, for apraxic and nonapraxic patients. Because of the labor-intensive nature of these observations, larger samples were simply not feasible. Within the limitations of sample size, the subgroups do not differ in the relative frequency of the individual movements emitted. That is, the proportion of flips, rotations, slides or pick-ups of blocks is approximately the same for all groups. What does appear to characterize manually apraxic patients working on constructional tasks, is the higher number of movements per event, such as placement of a block (regardless of whether the placement is correct or not). Manual apraxics emit almost as many individual movements over a constant time period as do other patients, but their proportion of completed acts is lower. This is consistent with the idea that it is the *selection* of appropriate movements which is particularly affected in apraxia (Kimura, 1979), rather than either movement repertoire or motility.

Relation to visuoperceptual disorders

A corollary of the suggestion that the right hemisphere contributes important visuoperceptual components to constructional ability, is that performance on visuoperceptual tasks should be more highly related to constructional disability in patients with right-hemisphere lesions than in patients with left lesions (deRenzi & Faglioni, 1967). It is very difficult to evaluate this claim because such a relationship might simply be an artifact of the greater incidence of perceptual deficits after right-hemisphere damage. Impairment has been reported after right-sided lesions for even quite basic perceptual processes, with little or no constructional component. Some examples are identifying the orientation of a line (Benton, Hannay, & Varney, 1975), enumerating a group of dots, identifying line drawings of nonsense designs (Kimura, 1963), and fusing stereoscopic images (Carmon & Bechtoldt, 1969; Benton & Hècaen, 1970; Stokes & Kimura, 1992).

In an attempt to determine more precisely the types of perceptual tasks which contribute to visuoconstructional disability, Dr. Larry Leach[2] in the present author's laboratory presented two perceptual tasks, a matrix-identification task, and a stereograms task. The matrix task was simply a series of 3 × 3 black-and-white designs (intended to resemble the Block Design patterns), each presented briefly. Then a second design was presented, and the patient was required to point out which of the nine block-squares had been changed (a variation on a task devised by Warrington & James, 1967). Although patients with right-hemisphere lesions were indeed somewhat worse than patients with left-hemisphere lesions, the difference was not large. Moreover, the relation to Block Design scores was not impressive in either group.

However, performance on the stereograms was significantly related to Block Design scores. A series of 20 Julesz-type cards was presented in a standard stereoscope, four examples each of five different figures (diamond, circle, etc.), in random order. For each stereoscopic stimulus, the patient identified it by pointing to the corresponding drawing on a card containing all the figures. This procedure was used to ensure that most aphasic patients could be tested. The stereo series was preceded by a series of "mock" stereograms in identical positions, in which a raised cut-out was actually pasted on the cards. On this mock series, all patients (16 with right-hemisphere lesions, and 16 with left-hemisphere lesions, fairly matched for extent of damage) identified all items

Table 7.9 Stereograms and Block Design scores

Group	*N*	Stereograms (max. = 20)	Block Design (max. = 48)	
Left lesions	16	19.6 (1.5)	20.8 (9.2)	
Right lesions	16	16.8 (5.2)	24.1 (14.9)	
No errors on stereo	10	—	33.7 (8.6)	$p < .001$
Errors on stero	6	—	8.0 (6.3)	

correctly. Yet on the stereograms series, six of the patients with right-hemisphere lesions made some errors, while only one of the left-lesioned patients made any errors ($\chi^2 = 4.67$, df = 1, $p < .04$). This would be expected in view of previous research (Carmon & Bechtoldt, 1969; Benton & Hècaen, 1970).

What was striking, however, was the very close relation, in the right-hemisphere group, between stereogram scores and Block Design scores. The Pearson *r*-correlation between these scores was .75 (df = 14, $p < .01$), suggesting that some common factor is responsible for over 50% of the variance on the two tests. Moreover, when the patients were divided into two groups on the basis of their stereogram performance (Table 7.9), their Block Design scores were also extremely divergent. It should be pointed out that the Block Design and stereogram tests were administered by different examiners.

Without information on other basic perceptual functions, it is not possible to know whether some ability related to depth perception is critical, or whether a range of perceptual functions must be affected, for visuo-constructive ability to be impaired. Four of the six patients impaired on stereograms had been administered an abbreviated series of Mooney Closure Figures, and their scores were extremely low (0, 0, 1, 4 out of a possible 13). Thus, all but one of the four scored about a standard deviation below the already low mean for patients with right-hemisphere lesions (Kimura, 1986). It may be, therefore, that extremely poor constructional ability is associated in right-sided lesions with generalized visuoperceptual deficits.

These results are suggestive, but we must caution that with the present sample size, the apparent relation between visuoperceptual and constructional ability may be due to pathology which coincidentally affects two systems, both of which are significantly right-hemisphere dependent. Only by increasing the sample size, and by studying patients with more restricted lesions will we be able to determine the degree or necessity of the association between the perceptual and constructional functions.

No such comparison could be made in patients with left-hemisphere lesions, since they performed so well on the stereograms; but since their Block Design performance is approximately the same as that of patients with right-hemisphere lesions, it at least suggests that perceptual difficulties are not the main source of constructional deficits in the left-damaged group. As we noted earlier, performance in the left-damaged group is highly related to manual praxis. These combined findings do provide support for the idea that the right hemisphere contributes a perceptual, and the left hemisphere an executive component to constructional ability, as originally suggested (Piercy & co-workers, 1960). Which particular perceptual/spatial functions are critical can only be answered by more studies of this kind.

Summary

Visuoconstructional disorders may occur with equal frequency after either left- or right-hemisphere pathology. They are closely associated with manual apraxic difficulties after left-sided damage, and with visual perceptual problems after right-sided damage. Constructionally apraxic patients with left-sided pathology show the same repertoire of motor responses in handling manipulanda as do unimpaired patients, but they emit more of such movements in completing an act. This finding is consistent with the suggestion that their difficulties are related to limitations in selecting appropriate movements, rather than in motility or in movement repertoire.

Notes

1. I am grateful to Rob Faust for painstaking scoring of these movements.
2. I am indebted to Dr. Larry Leach for collecting these data.

8. Manual sign language

Manual communication systems have sometimes coexisted with a vocal system, as in some North American Indian tribes and Australian aboriginal groups. In such cases, they served a variety of purposes—as silent hunting messages when sounds would be disruptive, for facilitating trade, or to circumvent social sanctions against speaking, such as existed during periods of mourning. Since such manual communication systems were never the major language for any of these groups, and were limited in their usage, they usually remained fairly elementary "pidgin" systems. Even so, they did not always merely represent elements of the spoken languages (Umiker-Sebeok & Sebeok, 1978).

More elaborate systems of manual communication developed almost exclusively among the deaf, where they have apparently flourished in every culture, despite disapproval from the hearing population, and often outright suppression from the hearing educators of the deaf. The pervasiveness with which idiosyncratic manual communication systems develop when even a small number of deaf persons reside near each other, indicates that manual/brachial movements form a very natural and readily available means of communication in humans. It has in fact been suggested that a manual system of communication long antedated the vocal system in hominids (Hewes, 1973, and see Chapter 1).

Manual sign languages, because of their visible nature, provide an excellent opportunity to study the interface between the structure of "language" and its motor expression, a relation much less accessible in oral languages. By far the most studied manual sign system is the American Sign Language (ASL). It appears to have been adopted by preexisting diverse signing communities in the United States, as an amalgam with the French Sign Language brought to this continent by two French sign-language educators (Woodward, 1978). As in any other natural language, there are many variants, both in terms of local dialects, and in terms of more and less formal usage (Fischer, 1978).

In ASL, the prevalent form of signing consists of unilateral or bilateral series of movements usually involving the whole arm. Typically, a particular hand shape is moved through a pattern in a location specified with respect to the body. For example, "pretty" is represented by one hand making a circular movement around the face (in a clockwise direction as seen by the viewer), with the hand beginning the movement with all fingertips touching, then opening wide as it goes around the face, and ending with fingertips in contact with each other again (see

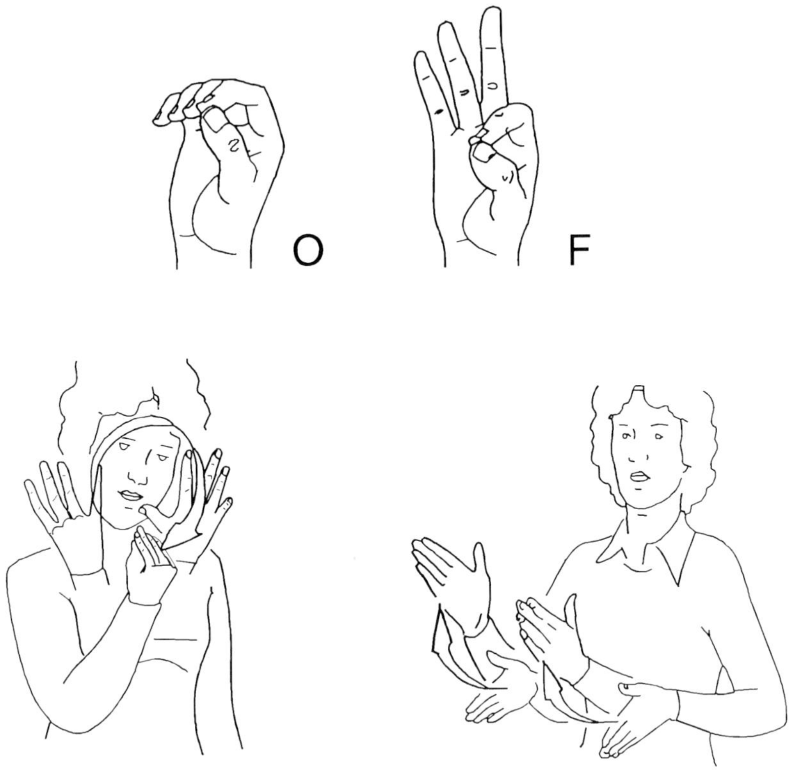

pretty let, allow

Fig. 8.1 (Top) Hand postures for finger-spelling "of". (Bottom) Signs in ASL for depicting "pretty", and "let, allow." (Reproduced from T. J. O'Rourke, *A basic vocabulary: American Sign Language for parents and children,* by permission of T. J. Publishers Inc.)

Fig. 8.1). Each sign roughly corresponds to a concept such as a thing or an event, but there is not necessarily an exact equivalence with English words or with words of any spoken language.

A native sign language like ASL is thus quite different from a manual depiction of a spoken language. "Signed English", for example, taught in many schools for the deaf, is a signed version of English which maintains English word order, and includes signs for inflections like "ing" or for the plural. There are no equivalent inflectional *endings* in ASL, such meanings being conveyed by the context, or by concurrent inflection. "Fingerspelling" is an even more literal rendering of a spoken language, being a letter-by-letter transcription, or spelling, of a spoken language into hand postures. For example, "F" is represented by a hand with the index finger resting against the thumb, the other fingers straight up and fully extended. "O" is represented by all four fingertips touching the thumb in an O shape. The word "of" is translated by the appropriate sequence, O, F. In this representation of a spoken language, movements are restricted to the digits, with the arm held relatively stationary. It is used during natural signing only to introduce a new, often technical term, or to spell someone's name for the first time.

There are claimed to be four distinguishing features of a manual sign, which when specified, will define it uniquely: (1) hand posture, (2) hand/arm orientation with respect to the body, (3) location on the body, (4) movement (Stokoe, Casterline, & Croneberg, 1965; Stokoe, 1980). For example, the sign for "allow" employs: (1) a hand posture in which the four fingers are extended and touching each other, and the thumb is extended slightly away from the hand, its tip not touching it; (2) the hands are oriented parallel to each other and to the vertical axis of the body; (3) they are located in the thoracic region just above the waist; (4) the movement takes them from a position in which the fingertips are pointing just slightly toward the floor, to one in which they are pointing slightly upward, thus primarily a movement of the wrist, but also of the entire arm forward. Many signs may employ this same hand posture, but in different orientations or locations, or with different movements. A similar statement could be made for each individual feature of the sign. It is the unique combination of these features which identifies the sign "allow."

Many hearing people who have no familiarity with a manual sign language still believe that there is such a thing as a "universal" signing system, that signs are largely elaborations of obvious pantomime, and that sign languages are thus rather crude and limited ways of communicating. A moment's thought should make clear that a manual signing system could no more be universal than a speaking system could be. Much of the research demonstrating the complexity, range, and sophistication of ASL has been done in Ursula Bellugi's laboratory (see Klima & Bellugi, 1979). While we must expect that a visual-motor language will have characteristics differing from an auditory-motor language, it is clear that ASL has grammar, syntax, and a rich inflectional system, making it capable of conveying any concept which an auditory language can (except perhaps sound!). In fact, its visual nature means that some ideas can be simultaneously conveyed in manual signing, which could only be sequentially conveyed by speech. Describing further the details and subtlety of the language are beyond the scope of this chapter, but the Klima and Bellugi book is recommended for a more complete analysis.

Neural mechanisms in arm and hand control

A study of motor systems in nonhuman primates has shown that corticospinal systems control arm, hand and finger movements contralaterally, but may control arm and shoulder movements ipsilaterally as well (Brinkman & Kuypers, 1973). This means that the left-hemisphere corticospinal system can control proximal movements of both the left and right arms, but can control distal movements only in the right hand. The mirror image obtains for the right hemisphere.

In the monkey, so far as we know, the two halves of the brain are equivalent for motor control, but in humans the picture is complicated by an asymmetry of function between the hemispheres. Chapter 6 outlined certain aspects of motor control which are critically dependent on the left hemisphere. These were postulated as having to do especially with the selection of appropriate hand or arm postures without visual or other external guidance. When there is a deficit in making such selections (apraxia), it appears to occur equally in the two hands/arms.

The praxis system was thus hypothesized to depend on centers outside the direct corticospinal systems, but to operate through them. It appears that left anterior and parietal regions of the brain are important components of a system for organizing hand and arm (as well as face) movements, but that this "praxic" system or systems typically accesses the motoneurons through the corticospinal system. If a significant weakness is present as a consequence of corticospinal system pathology, the movements cannot be executed. However, weakness or paresis is not a precondition for apraxia; indeed it can be seen par excellence in the unaffected left limb, ipsilateral to the impaired praxic control system of the left hemisphere.

In evaluating the effects of central nervous system pathology, therefore, we must be careful to distinguish between a mild weakness, which will typically be present only in the limb contralateral to the lesion, and an apraxia, which will typically be present in both limbs. Moreover, because of the differing natures of distal and proximal corticospinal control of the arms, we must keep in mind that finger movements may often be affected contralateral to a lesion while more proximal arm movements are not affected. Where finger movements are affected, hand postures will of course be impaired as well. Thus if, as a result of left-hemisphere pathology, movements are reported to be affected primarily in the right hand, but not in the right arm or the left limb, one must suspect a lesion of the left Rolandic region, producing weakness rather than apraxia.

The relevance of this to the study of manual signing is that the manual praxis system is presumed to underlie the capacity to employ manual movements for communication, just as an intact oral-movement control

Table 8.1 Manual signing disorders in left- and right-handed patients ($N = 12$)

	Disorder after left-hemisphere lesion	Disorder after right-hemisphere lesion
Right-handers	10	0
Left-handers	1	1

system is essential for communication via speech (see Chapter 5). The suggestion throughout this book has been that the left hemisphere is specialized, not for language per se, but for the complex motor programming functions which are essential to the language systems we employ. The language and praxic functions are not identical, in that the left hemisphere is also critical for motor programming functions which have nothing to do with language (see Chapter 6). We also know that certain linguistic functions may be mediated by the right hemisphere (Zaidel, 1978, 1989; Joanette and Goulet, 1986). Thus, it appears that some linguistic functions, such as semantics, are shared by the two hemispheres. We will discuss this again in Chapter 11. Because of the preeminence of the left hemisphere for motor control, the *production* of either speech or manual signs is not one of these shared functions.

We might expect the characteristics of the motor programming systems on which communicative functions are based, to influence the nature of the communication systems themselves. Since humans have probably been using complex oral or manual movements as a means of communication for at least hundreds of thousands of years, it seems probable that the prelinguistic nature of the motor organization will have imposed some significant constraints on the linguistic systems we employ.

One way we can see such an influence is in the detailed characteristics of the signs in a manual language. A motor control system based in one hemisphere but controlling both limbs, would presumably have a high incidence of movements involving identical commands to the two limbs, resulting in mirror-image movements. Battison (1974, 1978) has noted that if both hands are moving in an ASL sign, they are nearly always symmetrical. (If you try making two different movements with the two hands, you can see how difficult this is.) Even hand movements that are spatially parallel, as when both hands move to the same side, require different commands to the musculature, and such signs are also relatively uncommon. In contrast, rapidly alternating identical movements of the two arms or hands should present no particular problems for a unilateral control system, and in fact such signs are quite common. For many signs, then, the second hand is redundant, and signers can often manage to sign with one hand when the other is occupied.

When the two hands are used differently in signing, they typically do not differ in the movement, nor in location with respect to the body. They may differ in orientation, but usually only in terms of a 90 or 180° rotation, as in clapping (Battison, 1974). However, the hand *postures* are frequently different, usually with one hand stationary and the other moving. The stationary hand is typically in one of two or three simple hand postures. The neuroanatomic evidence we reviewed earlier suggests that we have more independent or disparate control for the distal musculature of the two sides, especially the fingers, than we do for the proximal musculature. This might make it easier for the hand postures to diverge than would be the case for the proximal muscles.

The motor programming system vested in the left hemisphere of humans, although exerting bilateral control, might nevertheless be expected to slightly advantage the right hand. It seems reasonable to think that the left-hemisphere-based praxis system has somewhat readier access to corticospinal systems in the same hemisphere with direct control over that hand, whereas access to the left hand may require additional synapses or at least a commissural connection. We suggest in Chapter 9 that this could, in fact, be the basis for the prevalent right-hand preference which we humans show as a species. In manual signing as well, if only one hand moves (the other being stationary and supportive), there is typically a preference for the right hand to be the moving hand. There appear to be no signs in which the hands change movement roles. However, signers can readily make the reversal and sign with the nonpreferred hand, though personal observation suggests that they do so with some awkwardness and reduced fluidity.

In hearing persons, right-hand preference does not manifest itself in better isolated finger movements of the right hand. In fact, such movements can be made slightly better with the left hand than the right (Kimura & Vanderwolf, 1970). It may be that the left-hemisphere selection system is less critical for finger movements than for wrist and elbow movements, or that it becomes critical only when more than one posture must be selected. In this connection, it is of interest that although the right hand is preferred by most deaf people for *all* forms of manual communication including finger-spelling, the left hand is apparently more often preferred for finger-spelling than for signing (Bonvillian, Orlansky, & Garland, 1982). This suggests that the importance of the left hemisphere in selecting movements, including finger movements, may be somewhat counteracted by the greater ability vested in the left hand for *executing* independent finger movements.

Aside from these very basic characteristics of signing imposed by the constraints of the motor systems, there may be other more general characteristics of our language systems, which can be seen to advantage in manual signing because of the more visible nature of signing compared with speech. These have to do with the selection aspects of motor programming mechanisms dependent on the left hemisphere, and are discussed below as revealed by manual signing defects after left-hemisphere pathology.

Manual sign language "aphasia"

A critical source for understanding the neural mechanisms of manual signing is the occurrence of signing disorders after pathology to the brain. A review of all known sign language aphasics in the literature (Kimura, 1981) found that 10 of the 11 cases had pathology to the left hemisphere, while only one was aphasic as a result of right-hemisphere damage. That one case was a left-hander, as was one of the 10 left-damaged cases. While most of the 11 reports were of dubiousutility inunderstanding the mechanisms of manual signing, due either to inadequate information on the status of the sign language before or after brain pathology, or to inadequate information on the extent and locus of brain pathology, several of the cases did satisfy minimal criteria for inclusion. It appeared from such reports that manual signing ability was largely dependent on the left hemisphere in right-handers, just as speech is. One additional case of sign-language aphasia resulting from left-hemisphere damage has recently been reported (Poizner, Klima, & Bellugi, 1987).[1]

Early reports of signing-disordered cases assumed that the defect was specifically linguistic in nature, and was either unaccompanied by manual apraxia, or unrelated to it (Critchley, 1938; Leischner, 1943; Tureen, Smolik, & Tritt, 1951; Douglass & Richardson, 1959). In most cases, this assumption was not adequately tested. In Leischner's case, only actual manipulation of real objects was assessed and found unaffected, but this is often true also in manually apraxic subjects, suggesting that it is the least sensitive of the various methods of testing for manual apraxia (see Chapter 6). In a later case studied by Sarno, Swisher, and Sarno (1969), ability to imitate the familiar movements of using a toothbrush, hammering, and so on, was assessed and found adequate. Again, however, such overpractised movements may often be relatively spared, when less familiar movements are affected, as discussed in Chapter 6.

In contrast, a series of unfamiliar movements (Movement Copying), demonstrably sensitive to manual apraxia, was found to be poorly copied by a patient with sign-language aphasia (Kimura, Battison, & Lubert, 1976), compared to age-matched normal deaf signers. The deaf signers also denied any linguistic content in the movements presented. This suggests that the defect in the aphasic signer was not limited to linguistic movements. A subsequent case report which employed similar movements for assessment of nonlinguistic motor control confirmed this suggestion (Chiarello, Knight, & Mandel, 1982). In both the Kimura and coworkers and the Chiarello and coworker cases, ability to perform familiar practised movements, such as showing how to use a comb or scissors, was minimally if at all affected. This supports the suggestion made in Chapter 6 that such movements are not maximally sensitive to apraxia.

Later reports claim to find no deficit in copying nonlinguistic movements in at least one of three cases of signing aphasia (Poizner, Klima, & Bellugi, 1987). However, since the least impaired of the three was the same case earlier found to be manually apraxic by Kimura and coworkers, there is some question about the reliability of the negative findings (see Kimura, 1990, for further discussion). At the very least, it is clear that manual praxis is not usually adequately tested in cases of manual signing aphasia. The focus tends to be on the language deficit, and the assumption that nonlanguage movements are unaffected is typically tested, if at all, with very minimal procedures.

It thus seems probable that the signing disorders seen after left-hemisphere pathology are, in fact, manifestations of manual apraxia, in the same way that most vocal aphasias are manifestations of disordered control of oral-vocal movements. The apraxia would give rise to defective selection of movements, both within and outside of the linguistic sphere.

Both production and comprehension of signing are affected after left-hemisphere pathology, insofar as it has been adequately assessed (Kimura, 1981; Poizner & coworkers, 1987). This fact has been interpreted by some as demonstrating the linguistic, rather than the motor programming, nature of manual sign aphasia (Chiarello & coworkers, 1982; Poizner & coworkers, 1987). An alternative interpretation is that the system for programming of movements might also be expected to participate in their processing (Kimura, Davidson, & McCormick, 1982). Thus, perception of signing may utilize a system overlapping with its production. The perceived movements might be encoded into a system mediating intrapersonal motor space, rather than external space, the former being more dependent on the left, the latter on the right, hemisphere (Kimura, 1977, and see Chapter 6). It also makes intuitive sense that the comprehension and production aspects of a communication system should overlap significantly.

Right-hemisphere contribution to signing

Due to the important visual component in manual sign language, it was expected by some that the right hemisphere might contribute more to a manual language than it does to a vocal language (Poizner & Battison, 1980). However, we have seen in Chapter 6 that the copying of quite complex unfamiliar movements is not impaired by right-hemisphere pathology, even when the latter results in gross left-sided neglect and spatial difficulties. This indicates that such manual movements are processed by a quite different system from that which processes other visuospatial information, presumably overlapping extensively with the system for selecting the movements, in the left hemisphere. From this point of view, right-hemisphere abnormality would not be expected to have any more effect on manual signing ability than it does on manual praxis for nonlinguistic movements.

In accordance with this expectation, a deaf woman with a moderately severe right-hemisphere stroke was reported to have had no signing difficulty at any time after her stroke (Kimura, Davison, & McCormick, 1982). This was true for comprehension of signing as well as for production. Later cases of native signers with right-hemisphere pathology confirmed the lack of signing difficulty (Poizner, Klima, & Bellugi, 1987). The latter especially noted that, despite the appearance of left-sided neglect on drawing pictures in two of the patients with right-hemisphere damage, they used the left side of space appropriately when engaging in manual signing. This is in accord with findings that copying of complex nonlinguistic movements by hearing persons with right-hemisphere pathology and left-sided neglect, shows no apparent difficulty with movements, some of which are presented to the left of the midline (Chapter 6).

The nature of the manual signing defect

The errors produced by patients with signing aphasia range from unrecognizable movements, through errors recognizable as a sign or part of a sign but unrelated to the target, to errors within linguistic classes. Perseveration is a common feature of signing aphasia, as it is in vocal aphasia. The fact that errors can occur within a morphological category, e.g., the substitution of another hand shape for the correct one, has been used to argue that the signing defect must be linguistic in nature (Poizner & coworkers, 1987). Other have argued that, although manual apraxia is present, it is a coincidental disorder unrelated to the signing disorder (Battison, 1978; Chiarello & coworkers, 1982).

Some of the confusion relates to an inadequate understanding of the nature of manual apraxia. It is clear that the common form of manual apraxia, ideomotor apraxia, may give rise to a range of error types, from amorphous unidentifiable movements, to movements recognizable as being in the patient's prior repertoire, but inappropriate in a particular instance. It is to be expected that, if a disorder in movement selection occurs, it will take place within the context of a patient's movement repertoire, which includes language movements. The fact that some errors occur within a movement category, be they linguistic or non-linguistic categories, is not necessarily an indication that the movement disorder is tied to movements of that class. We would not expect all errors, nor indeed most errors, to be a result of completely random selection. Only if there were unequivocally and reliably never any errors outside the broad class of movements being considered (in this case linguistic movements), would we have to entertain the idea that the movement defect is class-specific. So far, no convincing cases of this kind have been described.

It seems more probable that manual apraxia and manual sign aphasia are manifestations of dysfunction of the same system. Within this framework, the movements of language would be just one set of movements which are affected. We can illustrate with examples of perseveration, a frequent type of error in both manual apraxia and aphasia. When manually apraxic patients are learning the Box task (Kimura, 1977, 1986), requiring constantly changing hand postures (see Chapter 6), they frequently produce the hand posture which they used at the immediately preceding position on the Box. Patients who have manual signing aphasia also frequently repeat a sign which they have just used. Both of these examples might be viewed as instances of category-specific errors, i.e., errors within a limited domain of movements. However, both may also be viewed as identical errors in movement selection. Thus, if there is a dysfunction of movement selection such that an error is to be made, one movement with a high probability of being chosen would be the movement just activated, regardless of its linguistic or nonlinguistic nature.

Concerning other types of errors, Chiarello and coworkers (1982) have noted that when handshape errors were made by their sign-language aphasic, there was a tendency to substitute more common hand shapes from the manual language, for less common ones. Similarly, in hearing apraxics, when an error is made at a position on the Box task requiring the pressing of a bar by the thumb, a frequent error is the use of the index finger, one of the postures required elsewhere on the Box, and of course a very common handshape in all persons.

Apart from the obvious empirical parallels between manual signing and apraxia, it would be difficult to conceptualize an arrangement by which linguistic movements alone could be affected, without any deficit whatever in nonlinguistic movements. Such an extreme separation implies that language commands are entirely superordinate to their motor expression. We have suggested above that this is unlikely to be the case, given the motor programming constraints on manual signs. Instead, it seems likely that the linguistic and motor control functions evolved in an interactive manner, and consequently that the characteristics of the manual programming system are inherent in the language. It would obviously be extremely inefficient to duplicate the motor control characteristics in the language, that is, to have two separate systems, one for language and another for nonlanguage movements.

The details of the interface between the structure of the language and its motor expression will not be solved by an insistence that language is so special that it can never be understood by looking at visible behavior. We must remember that only overt behavior can interact with the environment, and thus it is the genetic substrate of *behavior* which is subjected to the laws of natural selection. Approaches to the study of language which ignore this, or take a linguistically solipsist view of communication are therefore unlikely to be productive.

Neuroanatomic mechanisms in signing

Since only a dozen or so cases of sign-language aphasia exist in the literature, and precise neuroanatomic information on lesion locus is not available on most of those, speculations about the specific systems involved must at this stage be tentative. Leischner's (1943) case was one of the earliest, and also one of the best documented, since the patient's brain was available for examination postmortem. There had been a stroke just prior to death, but this appeared as a fresh bleed and was relatively easy to distinguish from the old infarct which was the cause of the signing defect. The latter involved the cortex and white matter of the supramarginal and angular gyri, the same parietal region reported by Liepmann (1908) to be critical for manual praxic control. Tureen and coworkers (1951) claim that their patient's sign language aphasia was due to a left frontal tumor and hemorrhage, but the description of the degree of signing deficit through the various stages of increasing intracranial pressure is so incomplete, that one must regard it as noncontributory in terms of locus (Kimura, 1981).

Only two subsequent cases have had useful information on the neuroanatomic systems affected. Chiarello and coworkers (1982) claimed that their case also involved primarily the parietal lobe. However, there was also involvement evident on the computed tomography scan (Poizner & coworkers, 1987) of Rolandic and midfrontal regions. The patient's lasting hemiparesis, documented even two years after the stroke by Poizner and coworkers, suggests fairly extensive anterior involvement.

The only other case on which there is accurate neuroanatomic information within a reasonable period of the onset of pathology is also the only new case reported by Poizner and coworkers. She had damage to the left frontal, anterior temporal, and inferior Rolandic regions. There were also white-matter lucencies beneath the angular gyri and in the basal ganglia.

Poizner and coworkers (1987) attempt an analogy between the aphasia types in vocal language (and their neuroanatomic substrates), with those in the manual language. Thus, their case (Gail) with extensive frontal damage, was viewed as having a manual analog of Broca's aphasia. She certainly had a shorter phrase length than the other two cases they report (originally described by Battison & Padden, 1974, and by Chiarello & coworkers, 1982), suggesting reduced "fluency." However she was also tested by Poizner and coworkers less than a year after her stroke, while the other two patients were tested 2 years and 10 years after stroke. Since neuropsychological, including aphasic, disorders do evolve with time, and since both the other cases had originally had more severe and generalized deficits, comparisons across these three patients are somewhat misleading. Nevertheless, reviewing all the cases of manual sign aphasia in the literature, even given the limited information we have, does suggest that left parietal and left anterior (preRolandic) regions may be the critical areas in producing disorders. These are also the areas paramount for manual praxis, confirming the anatomic overlap between manual signing and manual praxis systems.

Summary

Disorders in manual sign language occur after pathology to the left hemisphere in right-handers. These disorders show characteristics similar to those of manual apraxia—bilaterality of the disorder, the generation of amorphous movements, perseveration, substitution of one movement within a category for another, and so forth. Moreover, despite the highly visual nature of signing, comprehension of signs is affected by left cerebral damage rather than by right. This is true even when right-hemisphere pathology results in gross left-sided neglect of space, suggesting that the processing of such movements is not achieved by the same systems representing external space. Within the limits of current knowledge, the neuroanatomic areas affected in manual signing disorders appear to be the same as those affected in manual apraxia. It is suggested that manual sign aphasia is in fact synonymous with manual apraxia, but that the apraxia in this instance is manifest in linguistic categories of movement not normally available in hearing persons.

Note

1. Two of the three cases of manual sign aphasia described by Poizner, Klima, and Bellugi had been reported earlier by others, that is, Battison and Padden (1974), and Chiarello, Knight, and Mandel (1982).

9. Adextrality

Throughout this monograph, discussion has focused on right-handed subjects, omitting left-handers, and has also disregarded other potential differences, such as those between men and women. We know, however, that there are variations from individual to individual in the way the brain is organized, at least for speech functions. In this chapter we will discuss how patterns of brain organization for speech and praxic function vary with hand preference.

The aphasia literature has from the outset been attuned to the possibility that speech representation may not be the same in left-handers as in right-handers. Early hypotheses, exemplified by Broca (see review by Harris, 1980), proposed an extreme divergence such that speech representation in left-handers was assumed to be the mirror image of right-handers, that is, that speech would always, or nearly always, be represented in the right hemisphere. The gradual modification of this point of view, as more cases of aphasia with left- or mixed-handedness appeared, has been reviewed elsewhere (Harris, 1980; Kimura, 1983).

Currently, the evidence suggests that, where there has been no early damage to either hemisphere to cause reorganization, speech is represented in the left hemisphere in at least 95% of right-handers, as well as in at least 70% of left-handed or ambidextrous persons. The most often-cited evidence in favor of this kind of distribution has been the result of unilateral administration of Sodium Amytal presurgically into one hemisphere in epileptic patients (Rasmussen & Milner, 1975). However, nearly all those cases had early damage to the brain, making it possible that the population is not representative of normal left-handers.

The present sample

Most patients had been given a hand preference test (see Introduction for details), on the basis of which they were classified as right-handed (dextral) or non-right-handed (adextral).

In the course of studying the effects of unilateral pathology on speech and praxic function in the present population, we tested 73 adextral patients with unilateral lesions. These cases were selected in exactly the same way that our right-handed subjects were selected (see Chapter 1), without reference to hand preference or symptomatology. They should therefore be as unbiassed a sample of adextrals as it is possible to obtain. Of the 73 patients, 13 had onset of pathology before age 10, and these patients are excluded from further consideration. Fortuitously, of the 60 subjects remaining, 30 had left-hemisphere damage and 30 had right-hemisphere damage.

Speech representation

Our data on the relative incidence of aphasia after left- or right-hemisphere pathology in adextral individuals with adult-onset pathology, is consistent with the position that the left hemisphere is paramount for speech in adextrals (Table 9.1). Of the 30 adextral cases with left-hemisphere damage, 7 were aphasic, while of the 30 with right-hemisphere damage, only one was aphasic ($\chi^3 = 5.19$, df $= 1$, $p < .03$). This indicates a higher frequency of speech representation in the left hemisphere than in the right.

Although there is a clear predominance of the left hemisphere for speech functions in nonright-handers, the incidence of aphasia is nevertheless lower after left-hemisphere pathology in adextrals than in dextrals (7 out of 30 adextrals aphasic, as compared to 131 out of 314 dextrals who are aphasic; $\chi^2 = 3.85$, dr $= 1$, $p < .05$). This is again consistent with past studies suggesting a lesser dependence of speech functions on the left hemisphere in adextrals than in dextrals.

However, we do not find a higher incidence of aphasia after right-hemisphere pathology (1 out of 30 nondextrals aphasic, compared to 3 out of 196 dextrals; $\chi^2 = .466$, n.s.). Both Conrad (1949) and Russell and Espir (1961) do report a higher incidence of aphasia after

Table 9.1 Incidence of aphasia after unilateral damage in dextral and adextral patients

Patient group	Left lesions	Right lesions	Total
Adextrals			
Aphasic	7	1	8
Nonaphasic	23	29	52
Dextrals			
Aphasic	131	3	134
Nonaphasic	183	193	376
χ^2	3.85*	.466 n.s.	4.81**

* $p < .05$.
** $p < .03$.

Table 9.2 Incidence of aphasia in penetrating missile wounds

Lesion side	Left	Right
Russell and Espir (1961)		
Adextrals		
Aphasic	12	4
Nonaphasic	14	19
Dextrals		
Aphasic	186	3
Nonaphasic	90	213
χ^2	4.75*	18.7***
Conrad (1949)		
Adextrals		
Aphasic	10	7
Nonaphasic	9	11
Dextrals		
Aphasic	175	11
Nonaphasic	163	238
χ^2	0.005 n.s	31.7***

* $p < .05$.
*** $p < .001$.

penetrating missile wounds to the right hemisphere of left-handed and ambidextrous persons than of right-handed individuals (Table 9.2). The discrepancy between our data and theirs may be related to the differing pathology in missile wounds as compared to strokes. A missile wound, occurring suddenly, may be more likely to cause disruption to a function, at least temporarily, than a vascular insufficiency, which allows an alternative blood supply to develop. A report of a high incidence of aphasia in left-handers with rapidly-growing tumors might be attributed to the same cause (Gloning, Gloning, Haub, & Quatember, 1969). Any type of pathology which results in sudden or rapid disturbance is more likely to permit the detection of bilateral or diffuse speech organization than is a gradually occlusive unilateral process. Moreover, both of the missile-wound studies included even transitory aphasias immediately after trauma.

Overall, disregarding side of lesion, in our sample there is a significantly lower incidence of aphasia in adextrals (8 out of 60 nondextral aphasics, 134 of 510 dextral aphasics, $\chi^2 = 4.81$, df $= 1$, $p < .03$). Previous reports of a differential incidence of aphasia in left-handers and right-handers have been contradictory and/or have not achieved statistical significance (Conrad, 1949; Russell & Espir, 1961). Presumably, as proposed above, if speech were more diffusely or bilaterally organized in adextrals, this might result in a higher frequency of aphasia in sudden or acute pathology. However, particularly with strokes resulting from gradual stenosis where an alternative blood supply is more likely to develop, the same type of organization could result in a reduced frequency of aphasia.

The lower incidence of aphasia in our nondextrals is more compatible with suggestions of a degree of bilateral organization for speech than with an exclusively right-hemisphere representation in a significant proportion (Rasmussen & Milner, 1975). Although Rasmussen and Milner attempted to control for the effects of early left-hemisphere damage in their analysis of Amytal-determined speech representation, it must be remembered that their patients all suffered from epileptic seizures dating from birth or early life, and that this may have affected cerebral organization for speech, even when there were no residual *neurological* signs of left-hemisphere pathology. Nevertheless, our data do not rule out the possibility that a small proportion of adextrals have speech represented primarily or only on the right.

If we leave aside aphasia and look only at adextral nonaphasic cases, comparing more conceptual verbal and nonverbal functions as represented by the Verbal and Performance scales of the WAIS (Wechsler, 1958), we see a pattern very similar to right-handers (Table 9.3). Thus, the Verbal IQ is significantly higher in cases of right-hemisphere

Table 9.3 Verbal and performance IQ in nonaphasic cases with adult-onset pathology

	Left lesions			Right lesions		
Patient group	*N*	Mean	(SD)	*N*	Mean	(SD)
Adextrals	23			29		
Verbal IQ		97.9	(14.0)		101.2	(12.9)
Performance IQ		95.0	(11.9)		90.7	(13.3)
Verbal − performance		2.9	n.s.		10.5	$p < .001$
Dextrals	201			234		
Verbal IQ		98.1	(14.5)		100.0	(15.0)
Performance IQ		98.8	(13.7)		92.7	(16.6)
Verbal − performance		−.7	n.s.		7.3	$p < .001$

pathology, and this is true of both dextrals and adextrals. Within the limits of these tests, it appears that verbal and nonverbal cognitive functions are organized roughly as they are in right-handers.

Manual praxic function in adextrals

The data thus suggest that cerebral lateralization for speech functions is not remarkably different in left-handers and right-handers. The chief difference is a slightly (albeit significantly) lesser dependence in adextrals on the left hemisphere. However, in right-handers, as we have seen, the association between speech control and the control of oral and manual movements is fairly tight. In contrast, to the degree that an individual is left-handed *because of* an atypical control system for manual praxic movements, we would expect the hemispheric representation for speech and manual praxis to diverge. Thus in adextrals the right hemisphere might be vested with manual praxic control, which lends to the left hand an advantage usually present for the right hand in dextrals; whereas for most of these same adextral individuals speech is apparently still controlled by the left hemisphere.

Previous literature on the lateralization of manual praxic function in adextrals consists entirely of individual case reports (see Archibald, 1987; and Faglioni & Basso, 1985, for review). The consensus of both studies appears to be that there is a slight predominance of reports of manual apraxia from right-sided lesions. The limitation of such case compilations is that we cannot know the factors which result in the selection of cases for report. Since not all cases get reported, some bias may enter into either the source, or into decision-making at the journal's editorial office. Consequently, we do not know whether the cases in the literature are generally representative of adextrals. Further noise is added to the data compilation by the fact that neither tests nor criteria for apraxia are uniform across cases, since they derive from different authors.

To determine to what degree manual praxic function is vested in the right hemisphere in our adextrals, data are presented in Table 9.4 on the effects of left or right lesions on the Movement Copying task. As for dextrals, the two hands tend to be equivalently affected when there is no hemiparesis, and the data are therefore shown only for the hand ipsilateral to the pathology. Of the 30 patients in each group, 21 of the left-lesioned and 17 of the right-lesioned group had been tested on this task. Looking first at adextrals only, patients with right-hemisphere lesions are significantly more impaired relative to patients with left-hemisphere lesions even when aphasics are included in the latter group ($t = 2.03$, $df = 36$, $p < .05$). It will be recalled from previous chapters that in dextrals, manual apraxia is highly associated with aphasia. Of the four left-handed adextral aphasics with left-hemisphere damage, three

Table 9.4 Copying Movements Score—ipsilateral hand

	Adextrals			Dextrals			
Patient group	*N*	Mean	(SD)	*N*	Mean	(SD)	*p*
All left lesions	21	18.2	(4.0)	265	14.9	(6.2)	<.001
Left nonaphasic	17	19.3	(3.2)	159	17.9	(4.1)	<.10
Right lesions	17	15.4	(4.4)	175	18.9	(3.4)	<.001
Normal controls (first hand)				18	18.8	(3.2)	—

are also manually apraxic, suggesting a significant contribution from the left hemisphere to manual control in these cases. None of the 17 right-damaged patients tested is aphasic, yet their scores are lower than those of left-damaged adextrals. When aphasics are excluded from the left-hemisphere group, the three manually apraxic cases are thereby also excluded, and the difference between left and right groups is enhanced ($t = 2.95$, $\text{df} = 32$, $p < .01$). This is of course exactly opposite the pattern found for dextrals, in whom left-hemisphere pathology has the more deleterious effect.

A two-by-two analysis of variance, whether done on all cases or on the nonaphasic cases only across groups (dextrals, adextrals) and side of lesion (left, right) yields a highly significant side by group interaction in each case (for all cases, $F = 14.619$; $\text{df} = 1.474$; $p < .001$). Thus, left lesions have the greater effect in right-handers, and right lesions in left-handers. This interaction is plotted in Fig. 9.1.

Subgroups of adextrals

There were almost equal numbers of patients who were left-handed and ambidextrous. Left-handedness was defined as performing all but two of the eight probe activities with the left hand (writing being left-handed). All other adextrals were designated as ambidextrous. Scores for the ipsilateral hand for these two groups are shown in Fig. 9.2. Overall analysis of variance shows no interaction of hand preference and side of lesion, and the pattern of results is the same in the two groups, that is, right-sided lesions have the greater effect. The difference appears, if anything, more marked in the ambidextrous group than in the left-handed group.

Familial hand preference was available in only some of the adextrals. For those patients in whom it was available, it was scrutinized for the

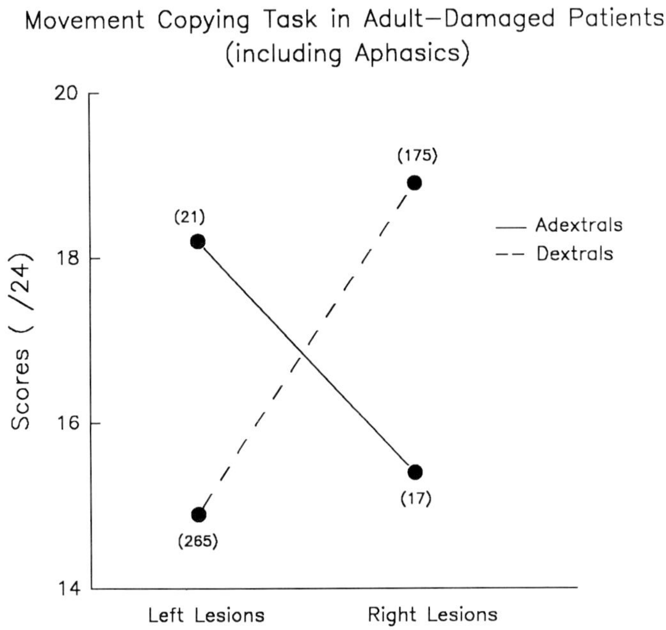

Fig. 9.1 Comparison of the effects of left and right lesions on manual praxis in dextrals and adextrals.

immediate family only, i.e., parents and siblings. The small sample sizes militate against any firm conclusions but the data in Table 9.5 suggest no striking difference between patients who have a familial history and those who do not. Both groups appear to show a right-hemisphere dependence for manual praxis.

Table 9.5 Copying Movement Scores related to familial history of adextrality

Adextrality present/absent	Side of lesion					
	N	Left		*N*	Right	
		Mean	(SD)		Mean	(SD)
Present	10	18.9	(3.3)	8	17.0	(3.3)
Absent	11	17.9	(3.1)	5	15.6	(5.8)

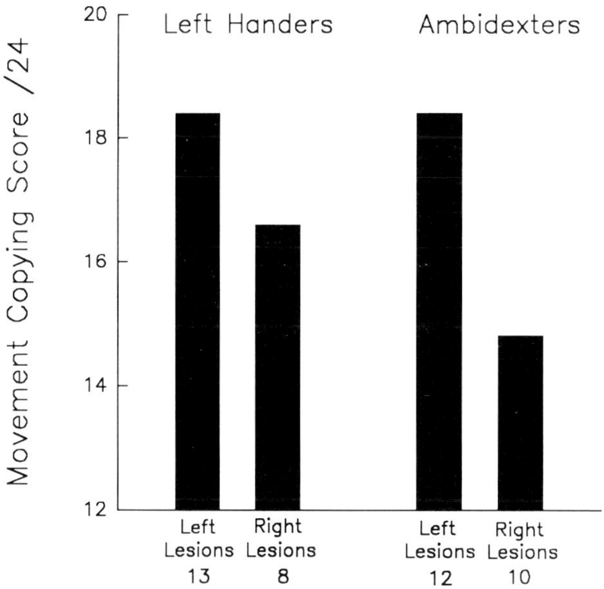

Fig. 9.2 Comparison of effects of left and right lesions in ambidextrous and left-handed patients.

Oral praxic function in adextrals

We have seen that, although speech representation in adextrals is significantly more dependent on the left hemisphere than the right, this pattern appears reversed for manual praxis. For the latter, the right hemisphere is paramount in adextrals. The question arises whether oral movement control will parallel speech control or manual praxic control. Because the oral-movements tasks were begun later in the series of patients than manual movements, the sample sizes are smaller, and statistical tests are therefore more problematic. Data for imitation of single oral and multiple oral movements are shown in Table 9.6.

As would be expected from the very tight association between oral movements and speech (Chapter 5), the inclusion of aphasics in the left-lesioned dextral group significantly lowers the oral-movement scores, relative to right lesions. When aphasics are excluded, there are no significant differences between dextral and adextral groups, nor any significant interaction of group by side. Nevertheless, there is a tendency for right lesions to have a somewhat larger effect on reproduction of *single* oral movements in adextrals ($t = 2.0$, df $= 25$, $p < .06$) than do left lesions.

Table 9.6 Oral movements

Group	Adextrals			Dextrals			p
	N	Mean	(SD)	N	Mean	(SD)	
Single oral							
Left lesions	17	15.8	(1.9)	276	13.7	(5.0)	<.001
Left nonaphasic	14	16.4	(1.1)	156	15.9	(1.5)	<.10
Right lesions	13	15.3	(1.7)	172	16.0	(1.2)	n.s.
Multi-oral							
Left lesions	15	6.7	(1.6)	222	5.0	(2.6)	<.001
left nonaphasic	11	6.9	(1.7)	125	6.6	(1.6)	n.s.
Right lesions	10	6.3	(1.8)	130	6.8	(1.6)	n.s.

The general picture which emerges for oral movements, then, is that they show a less divergent pattern between dextrals and adextrals than do manual movements. This might well be expected from the finding that oral movements are more closely tied to speech than are manual movements, since we have seen that speech representation does not differ markedly between handedness groups.

Implications for theories of left-handedness

The neural basis for hand preference is unknown. It has been suggested that right-hand preference is based on the presence of a motor-programming or praxic system in the left hemisphere (Kimura & Humphrys, 1981). This system, although controling both limbs as we have seen in earlier chapters, is presumed to have slightly readier access to the corticospinal motor system in the same (left) hemisphere, and thus to the right hand. If a parallel organization exists for left-handers, the right hemisphere should be critical for such praxic control, despite the fact that speech depends on the left hemisphere.

Some alternative views to the praxic interpretation of hand preference are:

(1) Left-handedness is the absence of right-handedness (Annett, 1972), and thus no major difference should be found between the effects of left and right lesions. This theory would fit reasonably well the data showing that neuroanatomic asymmetries found in

right-handers tend not to be reversed in left-handers. Generally, left-handers simply show lesser asymmetry (see summary in Kolb & Whishaw, 1990).

(2) Left-handedness is related to some special development of the right hemisphere for spatial (Peterson & Lansky, 1980; Kimura & D'Amico, 1989), attentional, or other function. Presumably in that case, speech and praxis both may still be vested in the left hemisphere, as they are in right-handers.

The data presented in this chapter suggest that there is a strong dependence on the right hemisphere for manual praxic control in most adextrals. This dependence appears to roughly mirror that of dextrals on the left hemisphere. For nonverbal oral motor programming function, dependence on the right hemisphere appears less than for the manual system. For speech functions, the left hemisphere is paramount, though not to the degree that it is in dextrals. In adextrals, therefore, manual and speech control appear to be more dissociable than in dextrals. This may have some implications for the everyday behavior of adextrals which has so far gone undetected.

It also appears that although some people may be left-handed through specially developed spatial ability dependent on the right hemisphere, this is not typical of the average adextral. We do not have information on purely spatial tasks, but the data on effects of right-hemisphere lesions on the Performance IQ (Table 9.3) do not suggest any greater dependence on the right hemisphere in adextrals than in dextrals.

The finding of a greater right-hemisphere contribution to manual praxis in nonright-handers raises problems for the idea that adextrality is merely a random consequence of the absence of dextrality. If that were the case, one would expect at most no difference between the effects of left and right lesions on manual praxis. The fact that adextrality is associated with a special dependence on the right hemisphere for manual programming indicates an explicit neural mechanism underlying adextrality.

Summary

In an unselected group of adextral patients without early CNS pathology, speech representation was more dependent on the left hemisphere than on the right, consistent with the literature. However, the argument is made that speech may even be more generally bilaterally organized in adextrals than the Amytal data suggest. Despite the evidence for greater dependence of speech function on the left hemisphere in our sample, manual praxic function is clearly more dependent on the right hemisphere. This is true for both ambidexters and left-handers. These findings raise some difficulty for theories of left-handedness which propose that adextrality is the random consequence of the absence of dextrality.

10. Sex differences in brain organization

Neuroanatomic sex differences

Morphologic and functional organization of the hypothalamus is the basic differentiator of male and female reproductive behavior. Certain parts of the preoptic area are larger in male rodents (Arendash & Gorski, 1983), and the ventromedial (Richmond & Clemens, 1988) and preoptic regions are known to subserve sexually dimorphic functions in reproductive behavior. Parallel morphological differences have been reported in the hypothalamus of the human brain (Allen, Hines, Shryne, & Gorski, 1989).

Outside the hypothalamus, however, reported morphologic sex differences in humans are minor, and have generally not been shown to have any functional relevance. One exception may be the report by deLacoste-Utamsing and Holloway (1982) of the greater width of the splenial portion of the corpus callosum in females than in males. This effect is present also in the human fetus (deLacoste, Holloway, & Woodward, 1986). Since the splenium carries fibers from the parietal and occipital regions in humans (deLacoste, Kirkpatrick, & Ross, 1985), the simple inference is that more fibers are available for interhemispheric communication between these regions in females than in males. The only study comparing directly a behavioral variable with callosal width is one by Hines and coworkers (1988), suggesting that verbal fluency was enhanced and language lateralization decreased, by greater splenial width in women. At present, there are no human studies linking sex differences in splenial area with sex differences in cognitive function.

Another structure which is apparently sexually dimorphic and which may have some functional relevance to humans is the hippocampus. It has been implicated in spatial learning in both birds (Sherry & Vaccarino, 1989) and rodents (Jacobs & coworkers, 1990). The hippocampus is larger in males than in females in vole species which are polygynous, and in which the males therefore traverse a larger territory than is the case in monogamous species. We have no information on the relative size of the hippocampus in human males and females, but to the degree that it mediates sex differences in spatial memory, it would appear a likely structure for sexual dimorphism in humans as well.

Background of studies in humans

Differences in the way the brains of human males and females are functionally organized was first suggested by Lansdell (1961, 1962) in the sixties. These early conclusions were based on rather complex and esoteric abilities (interpretation of proverbs, preferences for artistic designs), and the neurologic patient samples were small and incompletely described. Nevertheless, these studies presaged a number of more extensive investigations which came to essentially similar conclusions—that unilateral cerebral pathology apparently had a more deleterious effect on intellect in men than in women. The simple inference from this was that cognitive functions were more lateralized in male than in female brains. This hypothesis is still viable for some functions to the present day, though significant qualifications have been made in the lateralization story.

Much of the data on sex differences in lateralization of function have been based on IQ tests, and particularly on composites of subtests, typically a verbal and a nonverbal composite (exemplified by the Verbal and Performance Scales of the Wechsler Intelligence Scale; Wechsler, 1958). Since IQ scores are usually weighted for age, it is possible to make rough comparisons across different samples. However, local variation in IQ pattern, including sexual variation, is considerable, making use of IQ norms problematic. Consequently, researchers have resorted to using Verbal-Performance discrepancies and/or local normative groups to judge degree of deficit after unilateral pathology (McGlone, 1980; Inglis & Lawson, 1981).

The limitations of the Verbal-Performance discrepancy score have been outlined elsewhere (Kimura, 1987). In using local normal control subjects, there are other concerns such as the probability that, in the normal population, males and females may not show equivalent levels of all abilities; and that healthy normal subjects may not be the ideal controls for hospitalized patients with strokes or tumors. We have therefore used as "normal" control subjects a group of older hospitalized preoperative patients who subsequently underwent endarterectomy on one side to alleviate transient ischemic attacks (Kimura & Harshman, 1984). These control patients had no neurological signs, and no abnormalities on computed tomography scans. Their IQ averages were very similar to the Wechsler norms (Matarazzo, 1972), but there were slight differences between males and females, so that comparisons were in each case made with like-sex controls.

With such comparisons, the only significant sex difference to emerge was the negative effect of a right-hemisphere lesion in females but not in males, on two verbal subtests—Vocabulary and Digit Span (Kimura & Harshman, 1984). No other subtests or overall scales showed significant sex differences. The pattern suggested that there might indeed be a more bilateral contribution to certain abstract verbal functions or to immediate verbal span in women than in men, but that this was by no means true of all verbal abilities, nor was it true of the Performance tests sampled.

Lateralization of constructional and spatial ability

Constructional tasks are usually defined as those requiring manipulation or execution under visual guidance. Data on unilaterally damaged patients for the two constructional tasks of the Wechsler Performance Scale (Block Design, Object Assembly) are shown in Table 10.1. There is clearly no difference between males and females in lateralization of these admittedly complex functions. When aphasic patients are included, as is the case here, there is in fact no difference between the effects of left and right lesions, as discussed in Chapter 7. This is true for either sex.

One might argue that the abilities sampled by these constructional tasks are so complex, tapping several functions, that they are not the optimal tests for studying possible sex differences in lateralization of nonverbal function. More appropriate would be more purely spatial tasks, involving imaginal rotation in some form, particularly since the latter normally show sex differences in overall score (Kimura & Hampson, in press; Sanders, Soares, & D'Aquila, 1982). Data are

Table 10.1 Lateralization of constructional ability in males and females with unilateral pathology

		Block Design/48		Object Assembly/44	
Side of lesion	*N*	Mean	(SD)	Mean	(SD)
Males					
Left	182	22.8	(11.2)	22.4	(9.8)
Right	112	21.0	(13.8)	20.6	(10.6)
L–R		1.8	n.s.	1.8	n.s.
Female					
Left	103	24.7	(11.8)	24.2	(11.1)
Right	88	22.6	(12.3)	22.5	(9.2)
L–R		2.1	n.s.	1.7	n.s.

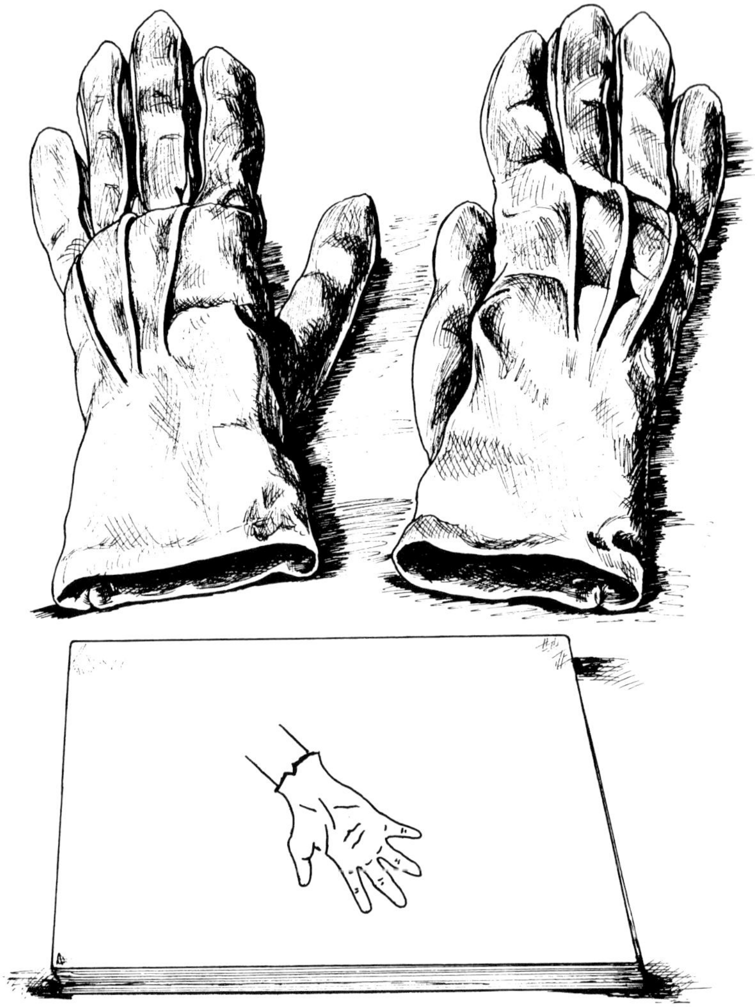

Fig. 10.1 Hands Identification test. Subject is required to point to the hand depicted by the line drawing.

available on two such tasks, which, because they were begun later in the series, involve a smaller group of patients than were available on the constructional tasks.

In the Hand Identification task, the subject is shown line drawings of a gloved left or right hand in various orientations, and must point to one of two stuffed gloves in front of him to indicate which is depicted (Fig. 10.1). No naming or any vocal utterance is permitted. In the Spatial Rotation task, the stimuli to be viewed are actual three-dimensional

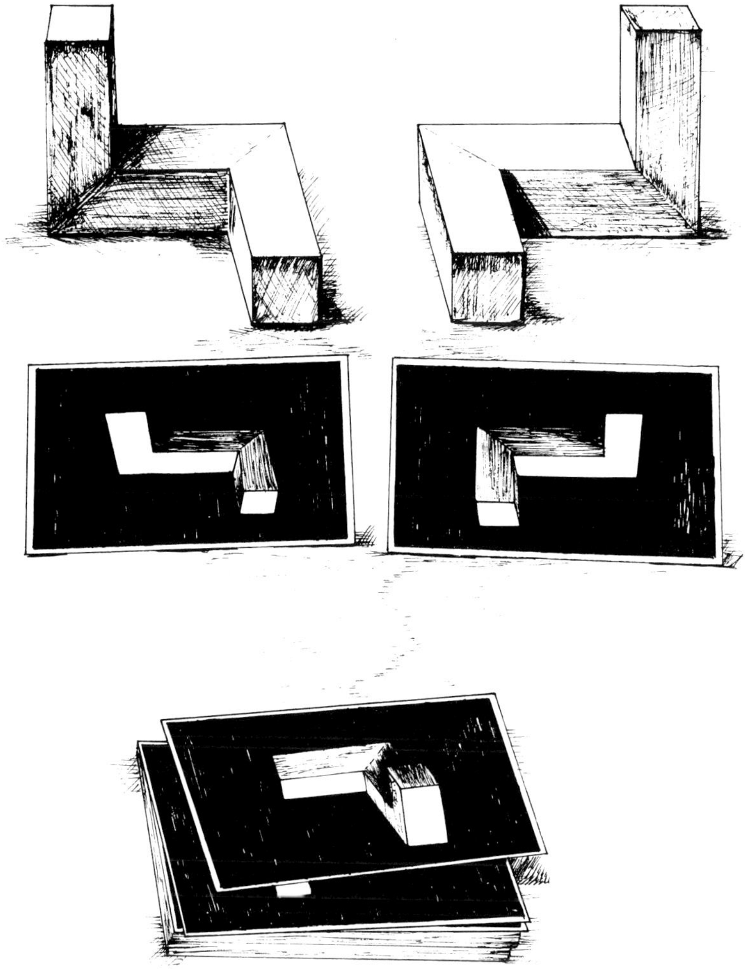

Fig. 10.2 Spatial Rotation task. Subject is required to place each photograph in front of the block depicted.

models of Shepard–Metzler-type designs. Two such mirror-image blocks are placed in front of the subject, and a pack of cards, each containing a photograph of one of the blocks, must be sorted by placing the photos in front of the appropriate block (Fig. 10.2).

In contrast to the constructional tasks, there is a significant difference overall between groups of patients with left or right pathology, as indicated by significant effects of side of lesion on both tasks (Fig. 10.3). There is only a slight trend for women overall to be inferior to men on the Hands test, but the effect of sex is significant for the other Rotation

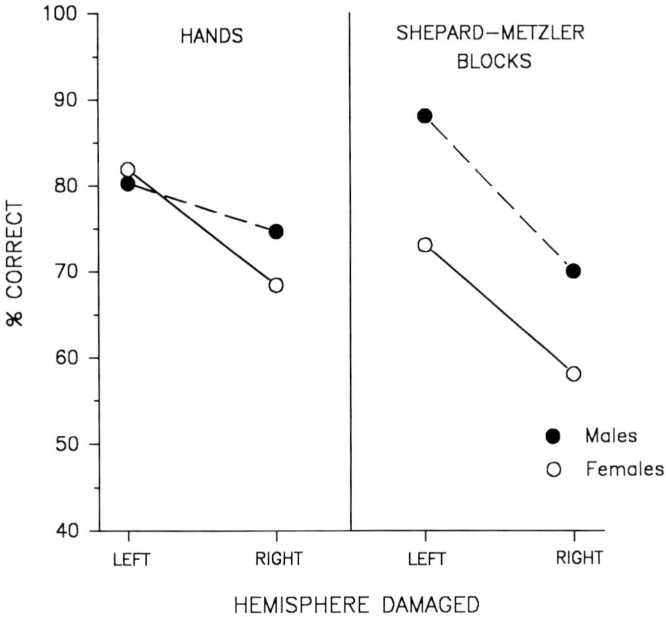

Fig. 10.3 Effects of left and right lesions on two spatial tasks.

task ($F = 10.38$, df = 1.56, $p < .01$). However, *there is no difference between the sexes in the magnitude of the right-hemisphere decrement* (in relation to the left), thus no trend for a side × sex interaction. It would appear that, even when sampling functions known to be sexually dimorphic, and demonstrably more dependent on one hemisphere, there is not necessarily any difference between men and women in the degree to which such a function is lateralized in the brain.

These findings would appear to contradict the suggestion from previous research, that the male brain is more asymmetrically organized than the female brain. Neuroanatomic findings of greater cortical thickness of the right hemisphere in male rodents (Stewart & Kolb, 1988), recently confirmed for overall volume in the human fetus (deLacoste, Horvath, & Woodward, 1991), would encourage the search for sex differences in functional asymmetry. Several studies examining perceptual asymmetry in normal persons, have reported a tendency for greater asymmetry in males (see review by (McGlone, 1980; Bryden, 1982). However, some of these apparent asymmetry differences must be reexamined in the light of our data on sex differences in intra-hemispheric organization (see below). That is, tachistoscopic and dichotic input (to visual and auditory receiving areas) might employ different or additional pathways within the hemisphere, in females as compared to males, to arrive at the critical processing systems. Sex differences in perceptual asymmetry may therefore not necessarily indicate differences in degree of brain lateralization. In addition, the possible availability of better interhemispheric transmission (via callosal fibers) might further reduce the difference between visual fields or between ears, in women.

Intrahemispheric organization

Speech

Evaluation of verbal intelligence in patient groups is typically made only in patients who are not aphasic, since the presence of a speech disorder is an insuperable obstacle to expressing ideas in the verbal mode. Males are, however, more likely to evince an aphasia after left-hemisphere pathology, and this fact also has been interpreted to mean that speech and related verbal functions are more unilaterally organized in men than in women (McGlone, 1980). Data on the present patient sample confirm the higher incidence of aphasia after left-hemisphere damage in males (97/200 or 48.5%) as compared with females (34/114 or 30%).

However, a breakdown of aphasic cases by locus of pathology (Table 10.2) suggests that the reduced frequency of aphasia in females is related, not to lesser asymmetry, but to a different intrahemispheric organization for basic speech function. Left anterior damage results in aphasia *more often* in women than in men, while left posterior damage is more likely to cause aphasia in men. (See Chapter 1 for definitions of anterior and posterior.) Since vascular accidents in our sample, when restricted in extent, more often affect the posterior than the anterior region, the systems which are critical for speech are generally less likely to be affected in women.

The higher frequency of aphasia after anterior pathology in women does not appear to be due to more severe or extensive damage. Incidence of hemiparesis in females with left anterior pathology (3 out of 14) is slightly but not significantly higher than in males (1 out of 18). If we compare only nonparetic males and females with anterior lesions, the difference between sexes falls just short of significance ($\chi^2 = 2.8$, df = 1, $p < .10$), but of course the sample size is reduced ($N = 11, 17$). Within females, however, even comparing only nonparetic patients, the incidence of aphasia between anterior and posterior lesions is significantly different from chance ($\chi^2 = 7.41$, df = 1, $p < .01$). There is no such locus difference in males ($\chi^2 = 1.69$, df = 1, n.s.), and the effect is in any case in the opposite direction. The combined χ-square shows a highly significant difference between the pattern of males and females.

Table 10.2 Incidence of aphasia after localized lesions in males and females

Group	*N*	Number aphasic	*p*
Left anterior			
Males	18	5 (28%)	
Females	14	9 (64%)	<.04
Left central			
Males	13	1 (8%)	
Females	10	0 (0%)	n.s.
Left posterior			
Males	46	19 (41%)	
Females	30	4 (13%)	<.01
Left temporal			
Males	18	6 (33%)	
Females	13	3 (23%)	n.s.
Left parietal			
Males	9	6 (67%)	
Females	6	0 (0%)	<.01

Similarly, the lower incidence of aphasia after posterior pathology in women is not obviously related to presence or absence of neurologic signs, such as visual field defects. Thus, in the left posterior group, 14 of the 46 males and 8 of the 30 females have a complete right homonymous hemianopsia, and this difference between sexes is not significant. Thus, there do not appear to be large differences in the pattern of pathology in the posterior region. Moreover, the incidence of restricted parietal and temporal lesions is almost exactly the same in the two sexes.

The suggestion that basic speech functions are *not* more bilaterally represented in women is further supported by data on speech disorders after right-hemisphere damage. Aphasia after right-hemisphere pathology occurs with no greater frequency in women (1/84 or 1%) than in men (2/105 or 2%) in our patient sample. Studies from other laboratories confirm an anterior/posterior sex difference in left-hemisphere speech organization. Thus, global aphasia, a severe generalized form of speech disorder, occurs more often after restricted anterior lesions in women, but after restricted posterior lesions in men (Vignolo, Boccardi, & Caverni, 1986; Cappa & Vignolo, 1988).

Within the posterior region, for the smaller number of cases where damage is restricted to primarily temporal or primarily parietal lobes, the difference in incidence of aphasia between the sexes is significant only for the parietal lobe (Table 10.2). Thus the sexual dimorphism in function appears most striking for the parietal lobe. This is consistent with the report by Mateer, Polen, and Ojemann (1982), that cortical stimulation of the left parietal region results in naming disorders more frequently in men than in women, while stimulation of the temporal lobe yields no significant difference between the sexes.

The question arises whether the nature of the aphasic disorder is different for males and females with pathology in equivalent regions. In Chapter 4, the nature of speech impairment after pathology to anterior and posterior, as well as more restricted areas, was described. Aphasia from anterior lesions was found overall to result in reduced fluency, and in relatively poorer reproduction of individual speech sounds than of multi-syllabic phrases. Aphasia from posterior lesions, in contrast, was found to be associated with adequate fluency, and with relatively better reproduction of single speech sounds than of phrases.

Table 10.3 compares the pattern of deficits in aphasic patients after anterior pathology in men and women. With such small sample sizes, statistical comparisons are not useful, but an overview of all the data suggests that, for both sexes, fluency is low and the repetition of single sounds is impaired relative to phrases. There are no suggestive differences between the sexes in this respect. However, the female aphasics across all tasks appear to be more impaired, and also to have larger variances than the males, with the sole exception of phrase repetition. This suggests that the anterior region may be mediating more varied components of the speech functions in females, and perhaps is doing so through more than one anterior system. With a sample size of nine, it is not possible to make a meaningful subdivision to test the latter

Table 10.3 Aphasics with left anterior pathology

	Males ($N = 5$)		Females ($N = 9$)	
Test	Mean	(SD)	Mean	(SD)
Receptive (/43)	40.8	(1.7)	30.9	(9.3)
Expressive (/47)	41.5	(5.9)	33.9	(15.9)
Fluency	6.6	(3.5)	5.4	(3.9)
Token test (/84)	63.0	(5.7)	54.2	(18.0)
Single speech repetition (/20)	15.0	(2.8)	14.3	(5.3)
Phrase repetition (/54)	50.0	(4.9)	51.5	(4.3)

Table 10.4 Aphasics with left posterior pathology

Test	Males (N = 19)		Females (N = 4)	
	Mean	(SD)	Mean	(SD)
Receptive (/43)	34.0	(8.3)	39.0	(4.6)
Expressive (/47)	37.6	(10.3)	36.8	(6.4)
Fluency	12.7	(5.6)	15.3	(7.9)
Token test (/84)	61.6	(16.6)	64.3	(17.3)
Single speech repetition (/20)	17.4	(1.8)	18.8	(1.0)
Phrase repetition (/54)	44.8	(10.4)	43.3	(17.2)

hypothesis. Only enlarged sample sizes in future will allow for such a breakdown.

Male and female aphasics with posterior lesions (Table 10.4) appear even more comparable than do the anterior cases. There is a slight trend for female patients to be less impaired than males, but the sample size of only four prohibits a strong inference in this respect. Both sexes show high fluency, and relatively greater difficulty in repeating back phrases than single speech sounds, as was earlier reported for the posterior group as a whole. Thus, although women are less likely to be made aphasic from posterior damage than are males, their pattern of aphasia is not strikingly different. This could be interpreted as further support for the idea that speech functions are not more right-hemisphere dependent in females, in that a more bilateral organization in women might be expected to result in greater qualitative differences between the sexes.

There were no females in our sample who were made aphasic by a lesion restricted to the parietal lobe. Thus, comparison with male aphasics cannot be made. Three of the four aphasic women with posterior damage actually had pathology to the temporal lobe, and it will be recalled from Table 10.2 that there was no difference between the sexes in the incidence of aphasia from restricted temporal lesions (but of course sample sizes for localized lesions are small). The question whether there is nevertheless a difference in the nature of the aphasia after temporal-lobe damage appears also to be answered in the negative (Table 10.5). With only six males and three females, we must be cautious in making inferences, but it is evident that fluency is high in both sexes. Moreover, the striking contrast between poor repetition of multisyllabic phrases and good repetition of single sounds is present in each group. Single speech sounds are repeated almost perfectly by all patients, male

Table 10.5 Aphasics with left temporal pathology

Test	Males ($N = 6$)		Females ($N = 3$)	
	Mean	(SD)	Mean	(SD)
Receptive (/43)	35.7	(6.9)	40.3	(4.6)
Expressive (/47)	36.7	(11.0)	39.3	(4.7)
Fluency	12.4	(6.4)	15.4	(9.7)
Token test (/84)	75.0	(2.8)	71.7	(10.8)
Single speech repetition (/20)	18.3	(1.5)	19.0	(1.0)
Phrase repetition (/54)	38.3	(14.2)	42.0	(20.8)

or female, but phrase repetition is more impaired in the temporal-lobe group than in any other group. There is also relatively good comprehension when no repetition is required, as indicated by the Receptive scores and the scores on the Token test.

It appears, then, that the temporal lobe may be organized for speech control in a fairly comparable manner in men and women. The anterior region also shows some equivalence between the sexes, but does appear to have more varied speech functions in women. The parietal lobe is clearly more critical for speech in men than in women, and one may speculate that some of the functions of the parietal region in males are in fact mediated by anterior systems in females. This suggestion will become more plausible when we look at the representation of oral and manual praxic function in males and females.

Oral praxis

It will be recalled from Chapter 5 on oral-movement control, that the ability to reproduce single speech sounds was very closely tied to the ability to reproduce single oral movements (Kimura & Watson, 1989). Thus, reproduction of single oral movements is impaired almost exclusively by anterior lesions, and in association with aphasia. However, reproduction of multiple oral movements was often impaired in patients who had no difficulty with the single movements. The multiple-oral movement systems appeared to be relatively independent of the single-oral system, and to be associated with those systems mediating fluency in speech. There was also a trend for the parietal region to be more critical than the temporal region for multiple-oral control.

Breakdown of data on single oral movements by sex does not look remarkably different from the whole-group data shown in Table 5.1

Table 10.6 Incidence of multiple-oral deficit (score of 4 or less out of 9)

Group	N	Number impaired	p
Left anterior			
Males	12	3 (25%)	
Females	12	6 (50%)	$\chi^2 = 10.82$
		12 (31.5%)	$<.04$
Left posterior		2 (9%)	
Males	38		
Females	23		
Left temporal			
Males	14	2 (14%)	
Females	10	1 (10%)	n.s.
Left parietal			
Males	8	6 (75%)	$\chi^2 = 6.07$
Females	5	0 (0%)	$<.02$

of Chapter 5, so the data will not be presented again. However, data for multiple movements do show significant sex differences, and are shown in Table 10.6. The multiple-oral task was begun later in the series of patients than were the aphasia tests (and has subsequently been modited), thus the sample sizes are somewhat smaller. It is apparent that the sex of the patient interacts with the locus of the lesion, in that females more often have a deficit after anterior than after posterior lesions. Males have slightly more frequent deficits after posterior lesions.

More informative is the breakdown into temporal and parietal groups. Patients with left temporal lesions, male or female, tend to show little or no impairment in reproducing multiple movements. With parietal lesions, however, there is a sharp discrepancy between males and females. None of five females have difficulty with oral movements, whereas six of the eight males have a deficit. Thus the role of the parietal lobe in multiple oral-movement control is seen to be critical in males, and the difference between temporal and parietal contributions is very marked. A test of the difference in males ($\chi^2 = 8.1$) is significant beyond the .001 level. The difference between these regions, noted in Table 5.8 of Chapter 5 is thus due to the male component of the sample.

Table 10.7 Incidence of manual apraxia (score less than 13/24)

Group	*N*	Number apraxic	*p*
Left anterior			
Males	16	2 (12.5%)	
Females	13	9 (69%)	<.01
Left posterior			
Males	43	19 (44%)	
Females	27	2 (7%)	<.01
Left temporal			
Males	15	2 (13%)	
Females	11	0 (0%)	n.s.
Left parietal			
Males	9	9 (100%)	
Females	5	0 (0%)	<.001

Manual praxis

Again, tests for manual apraxia were begun somewhat later in the series of patients than were tests of aphasia, so that the sample sizes are somewhat smaller than in Table 10.2. Manual apraxia is defined as a score less than 13 (out of 24), on a task requiring the copying of meaningless movements (Kimura, 1986). The score used is that of the ipsilateral hand, thus the left hand in left-hemisphere cases. Table 10.7 indicates that the occurrence of manual apraxia is more common after anterior lesions in women, and after posterior lesions in men. These differences are highly significant, whether one compares anterior and posterior lesion frequencies within males, or within females; or compares males and females within each region. Of the 11 female cases with restricted lesions and with manual apraxia, nine or 82% have anterior lesions; whereas of the 21 male cases, 19 or 90% have posterior lesions. It thus appears that the brain organization for manual praxis is even more divergent between males and females, than is brain organization of speech. (Recall that this is true for dextral and adextral subjects as well.)

Within the posterior region, there is again a sharp discrepancy between the sexes in the effects of parietal damage, but not for temporal damage. Thus only a small minority of temporal-lobe cases are manually

Table 10.8 Scores on Movement Copying (max. = 24)

Group	*N*	Mean	(SD)	*p*
Left anterior				
Males	16	18.3	(4.5)	
Females	13	9.7	(4.5)	<.001
Left posterior				
Males	43	14.1	(6.4)	
Females	27	18.8	(3.8)	<.001
Left temporal				
Males	15	18.0	(5.5)	
Females	11	20.6	(3.1)	n.s.
Left parietal				
Males	9	8.0	(2.8)	
Females	5	18.8	(3.1)	<.001

apraxic within males, and none within females. In contrast, all nine males with parietal-lobe damage are manually apraxic, even though only six of these are aphasic at the time of testing. (The remaining three cases had been aphasic in the early stages of their vascular accidents.) None of the five females with parietal damage is manually apraxic. The actual scores on the Movement Copying task (Table 10.8) are consistent with the incidence data. The most impaired subgroups are females with anterior lesions and males with parietal lesions. Thus the deficit in the group of males with left posterior lesions may be attributable primarily to the involvement of the parietal lobe, since temporal lesions alone have little effect.

These findings on manual praxis reinforce the suggestion from the aphasia data that those components of speech and motor control mediated by the left parietal region in males are subserved by a left anterior system in females.

Constructional ability

Performance on constructional tasks (see Chapter 7 and Table 10.1) are affected after either left- or right-hemisphere pathology. Insofar as manual praxis is related to performance on constructional tasks, one would expect that the brain systems in the left hemisphere which mediate constructional ability would overlap extensively with the praxis systems. Thus, females should be affected by anterior lesions, and males, if anything, more impaired by posterior lesions.

Table 10.9 Performance on a house-drawing task

Parameter	Mean	(SD)	Mean	(SD)	*p*
Left anterior lesions	(males, *N* = 7)		(females, *N* = 9)		
Number recognizable	7/7		5/9		<.05
Number details	7.9	(2.0)	5.3	(2.1)	<.03
Number lines	27.0	(10.5)	19.2	(8.7)	n.s.
Distortion ratio	.57	(.23)	.89	(.26)	<.02
Area (in^2)	8.0	(6.5)	13.8	(12.9)	n.s.
Time per line (sec)	2.8	(1.7)	3.4	(1.3)	n.s.
Time per detail	9.6	(5.8)	14.8	(10.6)	n.s.
Left posterior lesions	(males, *N* = 19)		(females, *N* = 11)		
Number recognizable	16/19		10/11		n.s.
Number details	7.5	(2.4)	9.5	(1.7)	<.02
Number lines	44.7	(39.4)	40.3	(15.1)	n.s.
Distortion ratio	.61	(.24)	.54	(.19)	n.s.
Area (in^2)	14.7	(13.4)	16.2	(12.7)	n.s.
Time per line (sec)	4.7	(4.7)	2.4	(2.2)	n.s.
Time per detail	18.9	(13.4)	8.4	(8.2)	<0.05

This suggestion receives support from data on spontaneous drawing, available for some of the patients shown in Table 10.8. These data (Table 10.9) were compiled in a retrospective review and scoring of drawings of a house, as part of a larger study on the effects of unilateral lesions on spontaneous drawing (Faust, 1983; Kimura & Faust, 1987). (See Chapter 7 for details.) Briefly, drawings are first scored overall as recognizable or not (assuming the target were not known); then they are scored for the number of identifiable details regardless of overall recognizability, the number of lines, the proportion of details which though recognizable are inaccurate or distorted, the total area, and so on. The time for the total drawing task is also divided by the number of lines and details, to give a rate measure.

Although the sample sizes are fairly small, it is clear that the sex of the subject interacts with the effects of a lesion in the anterior/posterior dimension. With left anterior pathology, females are the more impaired, to the extent that almost half of the drawings would not be recognized as a house if the target were not known. The proportion of distorted details is also much greater in females. Although the number of details is low in the female left anterior group, the actual number of lines is not significantly less than that for males. Both anterior groups, however, draw fewer lines than the posterior groups. That these data are not merely reflecting a generally poorer drawing ability in females in the normal population is suggested by comparison with the posterior groups.

In patients with left posterior pathology, the direction of the deficit is reversed. Now males show a trend for a higher distortion ratio. Males show significantly fewer accurate details, and take a significantly longer time per detail than do females with posterior lesions. It is also informative to compare within sexes across locus of lesion. Generally, the two groups of males are more comparable, showing only strong trends to differ in the number of lines produced, and in time per detail. Within females, however, those with anterior lesions show significantly lower numbers of details, as well as lines, and have a much higher distortion ratio.

Other typical constructional tasks require the assembling of pieces or blocks under visual guidance, and are exemplified by the Block Design and Object Assembly subtests of the WAIS (Wechsler, 1958). The data presented earlier in Table 10.1 clearly indicated no difference between men and women in the functional lateralization for these tasks. However, when we compare the effects of anterior and posterior lesions, sex differences again emerge (Table 10.10). Raw (unscaled) scores are used for comparison, since they have a larger range than do the scaled scores. An analysis of variance indicates that male and female groups do not

Table 10.10 Raw scores on constructional tasks (left-hemisphere lesions)

			Block Design/48			Object Assembly/44		
Group	*N*	Age	Mean	(SD)	*p*	Mean	(SD)	*p*
Left anterior								
Females	13	58.6	10.8	(8.8)		14.4	(8.1)	
Males	15	49.7	26.1	(7.0)	<.001	23.9	(7.0)	<.02
Left posterior								
Females	29	37.0	29.8	(9.8)		28.8	(9.8)	
Males	44	46.6	23.3	(12.1)	<.02	23.0	(9.8)	<.02

Sex: $F = 1.38$, n.s.
Sex × locus: $F = 8.37$ $p < .000$.

Table 10.11 Raw scores on constructional taks (right-hemisphere lesions)

Group	*N*	Age	Block Design/48 Mean	(SD)	*p*	Object Assembly/44 Mean	(SD)	*p*
Right anterior								
Females	14	50.9	16.9	(11.0)		20.9	(7.0)	
Males	12	54.1	26.3	(5.7)	<.05	27.4	(4.9)	<.06
Right posterior								
Females	20	35.8	29.6	(9.1)		26.6	(7.5)	
Males	18	44.4	25.8	(16.9)	n.s.	21.3	(11.9)	<.06

Sex: $F = .54$, n.s.
Sex × locus: $F = 3.78$, $p < .03$.

differ from each other overall, but there is a significant interaction between sex and locus of lesion. Male and female groups differ significantly from each other for both anterior and posterior loci, and on both subtests. However, while female anterior and posterior groups also differ significantly from each other ($p < .000$), this is not true for the males. Thus, the parallel with manual apraxia is weaker for males than for females, but the dependence of constructional ability on anterior regions in women is unequivocal.

Since constructional tasks can also be affected by right-hemisphere damage, one might ask whether the anterior/posterior feature of sex differences in left-hemisphere organization applies also to the right hemisphere. Table 10.11 suggests that it does. Again, there is a significant sex-by-locus interaction. Subsequent *t*-tests show the difference between males and females to be weakest for the posterior groups, especially on Block Design. Within females, there is a significant difference between anterior and posterior groups for Block Design ($p < .01$), with a strong trend also for Object Assembly ($p < .06$). For males the difference approaches significance only in the case of Object Assembly ($p > .06$). Again, there is no reason to think that extent of damage in the anterior region differentiates males and females, the incidence of hemiparesis, for example, being 3 of 12 men and 4 of 14 women.

One difficulty in making these comparisons is the variation in mean age amongst the groups. Performance on these two WAIS subtests is particularly susceptible to the age of the subject (Wechsler, 1958). In order to equate for variations in age, data are presented in Table 10.12

Table 10.12 Raw scores on constructional tasks (subjects over 50 years of age)

Group	N	Block Design/48 Mean	(SD)	p	Object Assembly/44 Mean	(SD)	p
Left anterior							
Females	12	9.3	(7.2)		13.0	(7.2)	
Males	7	21.1	(6.7)	<.02	20.9	(8.7)	<.07
Left posterior							
Females	8	22.4	(4.8)		20.3	(9.4)	
Males	24	19.2	(9.4)	n.s.	20.0	(8.4)	n.s.
Right anterior							
Females	9	11.9	(9.9)		20.4	(6.6)	
Males	6	24.2	(5.2)	<.02	25.3	(4.8)	n.s.
Right posterior							
Females	6	27.7	(10.3)		26.7	(7.0)	
Males	7	15.1	(18.8)	<.03	14.7	(13.1)	<.02

Sex: $F = .623$, n.s.
Side: $F = 1.40$, n.s.
Sex × side: $F = 1.44$, n.s.
Sex × locus: $F = 6.85$, $p < .01$.

for only those subjects over 50 years of age. This also ensures homogeneous groups in terms of pathology, since almost all subjects over 50 have had vascular accidents, whereas some of the younger subjects have tumors or focal epileptogenic lesions. It can indeed be seen that in almost all cases, the older subjects (Table 10.12) are performing worse than the groups as a whole (Tables 10.10 and 10.11).

The relationship of deficits to locus of lesion in older subjects, however, is not remarkably different from the total group. An analysis of variance with sex, side, and locus as factors, shows no effects of sex or side, confirming the lack of an interaction with laterality of lesion, as indicated also in Table 10.1. There is, however, a strong interaction of sex with locus of lesion, as occurred with earlier analyses. Despite the reduced sample sizes, males and females with anterior pathology differ significantly from each other on Block Design, and show similar trends on Object Assembly, regardless of side of lesion. The sexes do not differ from each other with posterior pathology in the left hemisphere, but there are robust differences with posterior pathology in the right hemisphere. Moreover, within females, those with left anterior lesions are significantly worse than those with posterior lesions, for all comparisons. For males, the difference approaches significance in only one of the four instances.

Functional significance of intrahemispheric organization

Normal men and women, at least in Western cultures, differ in a variety of cognitive functions. Males are better, on average, on certain spatial tasks, particularly those requiring imaginal rotation to solve the problem (see Kimura, 1992 for review). They are also reliably more accurate on targeting tasks, where a projectile must be launched or intercepted (Watson & Kimura, 1991). Females, in contrast, tend to be superior on small-amplitude motor skills, including verbal articulation, as well as in rapid comparison of stimulus arrays to determine identity matching (Hampson & Kimura, 1992).

It appears that tasks on which males tend to excel require accurate processing of external or distance information. To be able to determine the relative position of two stimuli, or to launch a missile appropriately, motor control must be meshed with such information. Females, in contrast, excel on movements which can be accomplished within personal space, making fewer demands on distance information. It is possible that the difference between males and females in anterior/posterior dependence for praxic and constructional function is related to the sex difference in cognitive pattern. Thus, if movements are to be integrated with distant information, it seems probable that they would be heavily dependent on posterior systems, where visual input is synaptically close. If, however, movements are primarily made vis-à-vis the body as framework, then reliance on posterior systems may be less critical. It is of interest, in this context, that male and female rats differ in their dependence on anterior and posterior systems for certain maze-learning tasks (Kolb, 1990), in a manner consistent with our human data.

The suggestion was made in Chapter 6 that movements within intrapersonal space were more likely to depend for accurate programming on the left hemisphere, than movements directed to extrapersonal space. A logical extension of this argument is that females are more likely to have developed a dependence on left-hemisphere mechanisms, relative to males, a suggestion similar to that made by others (e.g., Levy & Levy, 1978; Geschwind & Galaburda, 1984). It is difficult to know how to test this hypothesis in our population since, if

Table 10.13 Scores on movement copying

Group	Left damage *N*	Mean	(SD)	Right damage *N*	Mean	(SD)
Females						
Anterior	13	9.7	(4.5)	14	19.1	(2.2)
Posterior	27	18.8	(3.8)	20	19.5	(3.5)
Males						
Anterior	16	18.3	(4.5)	9	18.9	(2.6)
Posterior	43	14.1	(6.4)	15	17.7	(4.2)

we simply compare left or right lesions overall, we encounter the difficulty that intrahemispheric organization is different between males and females. In fact, the scores of all men and women with left lesions (or right lesions) on Movement Copying do not differ significantly, suggesting that there is no greater dependence on the left hemisphere in women than in men.

If, however, we compare the effects of left and right lesions restricted to anterior or posterior sectors, a pattern emerges which does suggest greater dependence on the left hemisphere in women than in men (Table 10.13). When the critical region is affected (anterior in women and posterior in men), the difference in magnitude between left and right groups is larger in women (9.4) than in men (3.6). This is reflected in an overall trend for a sex × side interaction ($F = 3.15$, $p = .078$), and a significant sex × side × locus interaction ($F = 12.47$, $p < .001$). No such pattern emerges on the constructional tasks (Tables 10.10–10.12), nor would it be expected, since they depend on *both* left- and right-hemisphere systems.

Summary

This chapter outlined how brain organization for speech and for manual programming and constructional function varies with the sex of the individual. The data suggest that sex differences in lateralization of function are relatively minor. A more compelling sex difference is found to relate to intrahemispheric organization of function. For women, the anterior region in the left hemisphere appears to be critical for speech and manual praxic function, while the pattern in males shows a more even distribution of these functions across the two brain sectors, but if anything favors the posterior region, particularly for manual function. For constructional tasks, which sample both right- and left-hemisphere function, the anterior regions are again the more critical in women. These findings may relate to sexual dimorphism in human abilities, with males generally having better abilities relating to distance information and females to intrapersonal space.

11. Hemispheric specialization for semantic processing

The term "semantic" comes from the Greek word *semantikos*, meaning significance. In English it refers to the capacity for a sign, usually but not necessarily a word, to have associative or categoric meaning. The common restriction of the term to the symbols of language prejudges the importance of language in the mediation of meaning. The great apes, which do not naturally have a communication system such as humans, nevertheless have a high level of semantic capability (see Chapter 1). We do not know the neural substrate for sign-referent ability in chimpanzees, for example, but it is unlikely to be based on left-hemisphere specialization for language. The existence of semantic function in the absence of humanlike language should indicate that the latter is not a prerequisite for semanticity.

Neural mechanisms in reading

One of the most significant findings to come out of the split-brain literature was to establish the extreme dependence of speech production on the left hemisphere. In contrast, speech comprehension can apparently be mediated by the right hemisphere to a significant degree. It appears to be comprehension at a semantic level which is most readily achieved by right-hemisphere mechanisms, while phonemic or syllabic-level processing is, like production, more dependent on left-hemisphere systems (Levy & Trevarthan, 1977; Zaidel, 1985). This fact has relevance for understanding some of the varieties of reading disorders resulting from central nervous system damage.

In adults, at least two distinctive classes of reading disorders have been described after central nervous system damage. One is a disorder in which the letters or groups of letters can be sounded out correctly, but the ability to form or recognize words from the cluster of letters is impaired. This type of reading disorder is called "surface dyslexia," implying a failure to go from the printed whole word to its pronunciation. In some of these cases there is also a "semantic access" dyslexia, indicating that the difficulty is in grasping the meaning of the word—that is, in gaining access to the category which the word represents (see discussion by Ellis & Young, 1988).

Surface dyslexia contrasts with so-called "deep dyslexia," another type of reading disorder. In deep dyslexia, the difficulty appears to be in identifying the speech sounds represented by the letters. Individuals with this type of disorder thus cannot accurately read nonsense words, but are more successful in reading real words, especially concrete words, despite their difficulty in transforming the letters into sounds.

Case study

Surface dyslexia can be illustrated by a case we have seen in a 63-year-old man who suffered from a metastatic tumor in the left occipitoparietal area. Although he had an average IQ and was not aphasic, he had extreme difficulty reading. He performed well below average on a test of reading words, yet could identify individual letters perfectly and could read nonsense syllables almost normally. Indeed, his approach to reading was to sound out the words, and he succeeded in reading most monosyllabic words in this way. However, with multisyllabic words, he was relatively unsuccessful. Examples of his responses are: *himself* spelled as "h-i-m-s-e-l-f"; *contagious*—"contact, contayge"; *eliminate*—"element"; *ethics*—"a thick, ethic." Sometimes, he would read the word aloud correctly without being aware of it. Clearly this was a case where the letter groupings did not evoke any corresponding whole words, and it was only through uttering the component sounds aloud that he could sometimes identify the word.

Deep dyslexia has been described in detail by Marshall and Newcombe (1980) in their famous case G.R. This patient was an intelligent and formerly literate adult, who generated many semantic errors when reading. Thus, for *act*, he would read "play"; for *close*, he would read "shut." Concrete nouns were most often read correctly, and so-called function words were the hardest. Thus for the word *for*, he would read "and"; for *be*, "small words are the worst." The extreme difficulty with such words, in comparison with concrete nouns, prompted a description of the syndrome which was entitled "*Bee* but not *be*" (Gardner & Zurif, 1975). Clearly, deep dyslexics can, without being able to process or sound out each individual letter, associate a word or semantic category with a configuration of letters. To some extent, they can bypass their phonemic/syllabic difficulty. That they can do so, and do so most successfully for concrete, as compared to abstract nouns, indicates that they have relatively intact semantic access. That is, the categories accessed by the letter strings are probably normal.

The existence of these two classes of reading disorders suggests that normal literate adults employ both methods in the course of reading. The more experienced the reader, one might expect, the more likely she or he is to bypass the individual phoneme in reading, and to go directly from a letter cluster or word-configuration to the word. Yet most people probably also retain the tendency to sound out words, particularly when they encounter unfamiliar words. That these two modes of reading may be universally available in people is also suggested by studies of reading disorders in Japanese persons who have sustained left-hemisphere damage.

In Japanese, two types of reading are typically taught. One is a syllabic system, in which characters represent speech-sound units, very much like the reading of English. The other is an ideographic system, in which characters represent whole words, things, or events, and have no reference to sounds, like the Chinese system of reading and writing. Several cases have now been reported in the Japanese literature (see review by Sasanuma, 1980), in whom left-hemisphere pathology has resulted in a deficit in the syllabic reading system, without significant difficulty in the ideographic system. This is despite the fact that the latter is more difficult to acquire. It appears that such persons can make a symbol-referent match when they cannot make a sound-to-word match. In that sense, they resemble deep dyslexics.

In both the Japanese syllabic-system dyslexia and in deep dyslexia, there appears to be a difficulty in converting visual signs to speech sounds, yet the capacity for visual signs to access semantic categories is relatively unaffected. This has led some authors (Coltheart, 1980; Zaidel, 1985) to suggest that phonemic dyslexics are reading primarily with the right hemisphere, which as we know from the split-brain studies, is able to read and understand well enough to pick out objects of a particular category correctly. Yet this same hemisphere is unable to process speech at the phonemic level at all well.

Reading in deaf aphasics

In persons who acquire reading entirely via the nonsyllabic route, then, we might expect left-hemisphere damage to have little effect on their reading ability. One such group of people is the deaf population. Deaf people, even those who are fortunate enough to attend good schools, apparently have great difficulty in learning to read, at least in the phonetic languages (Conrad, 1979). One suspects that this is because they cannot use the sound system we use when learning to read. The letters and letter groupings must appear as quite arbitrary symbols for the concepts represented by words.

However, when deaf signers become aphasic in the sign language after left-hemisphere damage, their reading ability appears to be spared, relative to other communicative function (Kimura, 1981). Information on this subject is admittedly sketchy, but several of the case reports state that reading is unchanged from before. Most probably this is due to the same mechanism which allows ideographic reading to survive left-hemisphere damage in the Japanese cases described above. That is, it is probable that the deaf read via visual letter arrays rather than phonemic-syllabic units, and this method of reading can be mediated by the intact right hemisphere.

Semantic categorization in aphasia

It is often assumed in the neuropsychologic and neurologic literature that semantic function depends primarily on the left hemisphere, and that it is closely tired to the language system. Claims for the primacy of the left hemisphere in semantic processing have been based largely on observation of aphasic cases. Such studies, however, have employed words (either oral or printed) as critical cues at some point in the procedure, making it difficult to dissociate the aphasic patient's verbal deficits from the semantic ability (e.g., Chapey & Lubinski, 1979; Grober, Perecman, Kellar, & Brown, 1980).

The proposal that semantic categorization is dependent on left-hemisphere language systems is made explicit by Caramazza, Berndt, and Brownell (1982) through the following schema, applicable to the processing (and subsequent naming) of pictorial material (e.g., cup):

(1) There is assumed to be a low-level perceptual analysis.
(2) Next is a modality-specific identification (e.g., handle shape). However, even this stage is assumed to tap into a language (lexical) system—that is, "the process of extraction from a graphic input of the properties that are relevant to the classification of an object as a member of a category . . . interacts with the semantic component of the lexicon in such a way that perceptual parsing is constrained by semantic considerations."
(3) There is then modality-independent identification which defines category membership, selection of the lexical item which specified phonological and syntactic information, and finally, articulation of the phonological representation.

However, in the Caramazza study (as in other studies of this kind), patients were required to perform two tasks demanding verbalization: to label a series of quite similar objects as either a cup or bowl; and to say "same" or "different" to a series of pairs of cups and bowls which differed in small perceptual steps. Anyone who has tested aphasic patients will know that the *labels* "same" or "different," simple though they seem to us, are extremely difficult for aphasics to deal with, even when there is no doubt that they can make the discrimination.

In a study on globally aphasic patients, however, Glass, Gazzaniga, and Premack (1973) found that most could use nonlanguage (Premack) symbols to communicate same–different distinctions, and to convey the negative. Several patients, although unable to name objects accurately, could convey such names correctly using the nonverbal symbols. The authors conclude that their patients "retain a rich conceptual system and . . . some capacity for symbolization."

Studies on split-brain patients suggest that the right hemisphere is capable of a high level of semantic processing (Sperry & Gazzaniga, 1967; Zaidel, 1978, 1989). Zaidel concludes that the right hemisphere has a rich semantic system, but an impoverished phonology and poor syntax. Consistent with this view, Joanette, Goulet, and LeDorze (1988) have described semantic deficits after right-hemisphere pathology. Thus, right lesions impaired word fluency when the category was semantic (e.g., "animal" or "furniture") but not when the category was articulatory (e.g., beginning letter).

Semantic categorization in global aphasics

To determine to what extent semantic categorizations could be made when no or almost no verbal system was available, we decided to study semantic function in patients with extensive left-hemisphere pathology and severe global aphasia (Kimura, Clydesdale, & Teasell, 1991). The study differed from most others in that the tasks we used *contained no verbal material*, nor was any verbal instruction given. This procedure was adhered to not only for aphasic patients but also for the normal control subjects and for patients with right-hemisphere damage. We were thus able to see how a person with practically no verbal system available perceived and categorized objects and actions.

Subjects

Patients were chosen for having extensive vascular damage to one hemisphere, with both contralateral hemiparesis and hemianopsia. They were at least 6 months poststroke, with a minimum of a Grade 10 education and under 70 years of age. Because the test procedures employed required fairly long periods of interaction, spread over several weeks, it was not feasible to have a large sample:

(1) *Aphasic patients* ($N = 3$, two male, one female) were chosen for the presence of global aphasia, scoring below the mean of aphasics on *both* the expressive and receptive components of the aphasia-screening test (see Chapter 1).
(2) *Right-damaged patents* ($N = 2$, both male) had equivalent extensive pathology to the right hemisphere.
(3) *Normal controls* ($N = 2$, one male, one female) were spouses of patients, matched for age.

Procedure

All tests employed a probe item on a card, and four choices arrayed vertically on a single sheet below (Fig. 11.1). The examiner pointed to the probe, then swept his hand along the array, indicating that the subject (S) was to make a selection from the four pictures. The *only verbal instruction* was "Pick one."

Subjects were tested in four sessions at least 1 week apart, to reduce carry-over strategies from one test to the next. Tests were given in the following order.

Perceptual tests

1. *Object identity.* A drawing of a familiar object was the probe, an identical drawing being among the four choices.
2. *Complex pattern identity.* A geometric pattern was the probe, with an identical one among the choices.
3. *Object rotation match.* A drawing of a familiar object was the probe, with a rotated version of this object among the choices (Fig. 11.1).

Semantic category tests

1. *Spontaneous.* (Fig. 11.2) The probe was an object, and among the four choices was one in the same semantic category. There were seven categories (e.g., birds, tools) with three examples each, randomly presented, for a total of 21 trials.
2. *Primed.* (Given at least 1 week later) To inform the subject about the categories without giving verbal instruction, S was required to sort 10 cards into two piles. Five of the 10 cards were in a target category (e.g., tools), each wrong sort being corrected as it occurred.

The subject was then given the same three trials of this category (e.g., tools) as under the Spontaneous condition. This procedure was repeated for all seven semantic categories.

Action/Function category tests

1. *Spontaneous.* The probe was a depiction of an action or function (e.g., digging, cooking), and among the four choices was a related action.
2. *Primed* (given at least one week later). In addition to the probe first presented, a second probe was given, to help clarify which choice was most appropriate (see Fig. 11.3). The task was otherwise identical.

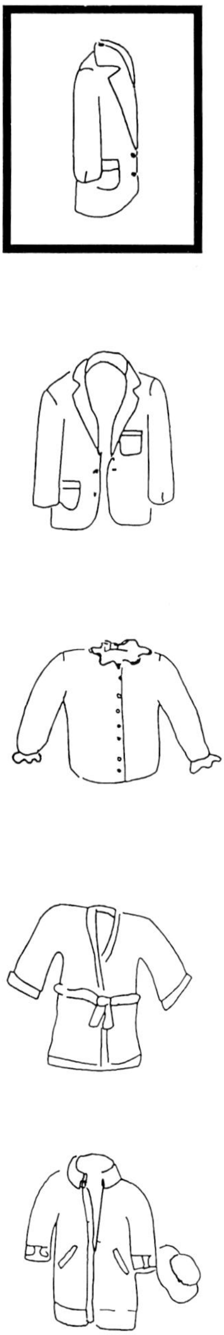

Fig. 11.1 Example of an Object Rotation item. The corresponding match is the first item below the probe.

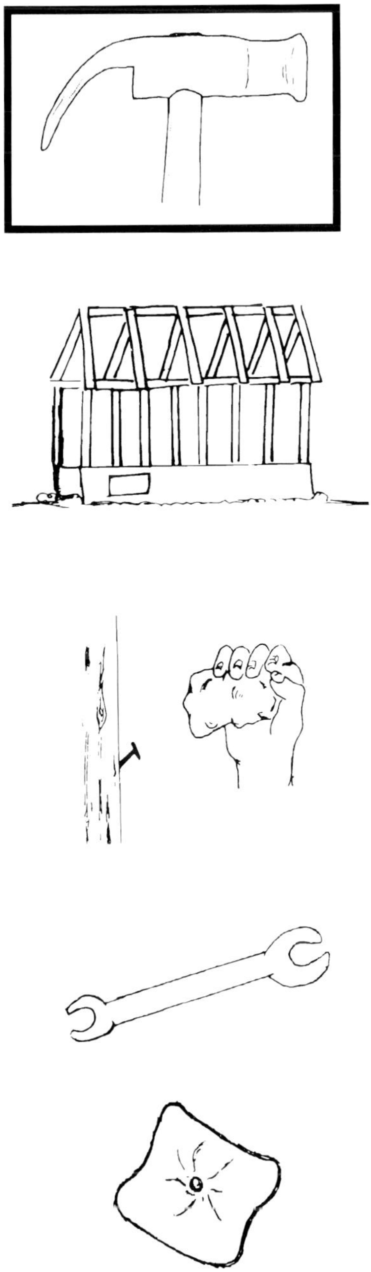

Fig. 11.2 Example of a semantic category item (tools). Choice of the wrench would be classed as a Semantic-Category response, choice of the house would be "associative."

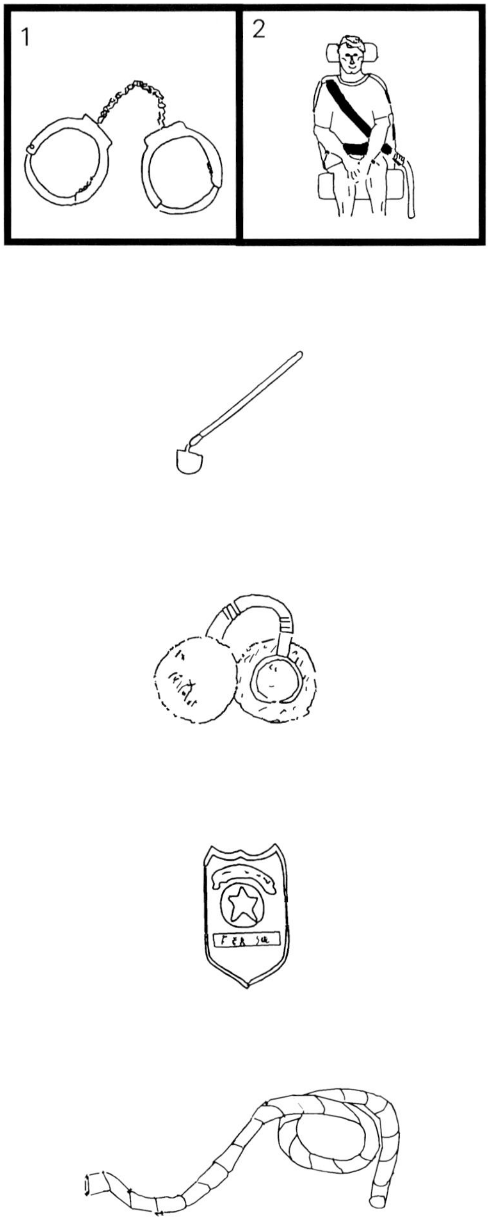

Fig. 11.3 Example of an Action/Function item. The card 1 would be shown in the spontaneous condition. This would be augmented with Card 2 in the primed condition. The rope is the intended target, choice of the badge would be "associative."

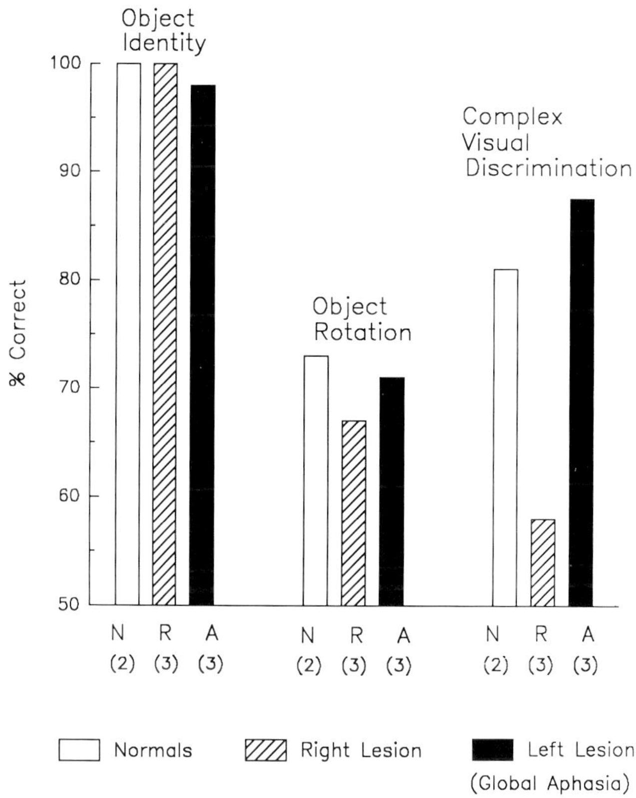

Fig. 11.4 Performance on the Perceptual tests.

Results

Perceptual Tests. All subjects chose familiar objects identical to the probe nearly 100% of the time (Fig. 11.4). On complex geometric material, patients with right-sided lesions made the most nonidentical matches, while aphasics performed like normals. When a rotated form of an object was to be chosen, aphasics again performed normally, while right-lesioned patients made slightly fewer appropriate choices.

Thus, the global aphasics were able to make identity matches of both familiar and unfamiliar stimuli, and to pick out rotated versions of stimuli.

Semantic category tests. Before priming, normals and right-damaged patients chose semantic targets below the chance level, while aphasics chose them above chance level (Fig. 11.5). Alternative choices included unrelated objects, visually similar objects, or those which had an

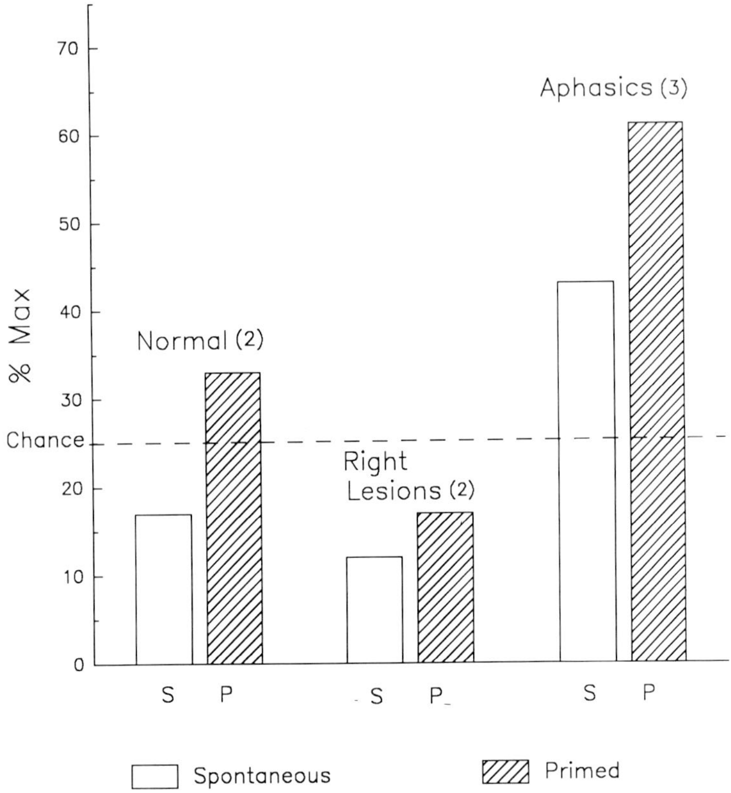

Fig. 11.5 Semantic choices on the Semantic Category test.

associative link (see Fig. 11.2). After priming, normals' semantic choices rose to above chance, and aphasics increased their semantic choices even more. Right-damaged patients' semantic choices remained below chance.

It was clear from the priming effect that normals could follow the card sort procedure which was used as a priming device at least as well as aphasics, but still did not favour semantic choices to the degree that aphasics did. Right-lesioned patients showed extreme divergence from other subjects on this task. It appears, then, that *aphasics favored Semantic Category choices,* both before and after priming, and made more of these than did the normal subjects or the right-damaged patients.

Action/Function Category tests. There appeared to be no significant differences among the groups in tendency to choose action targets,

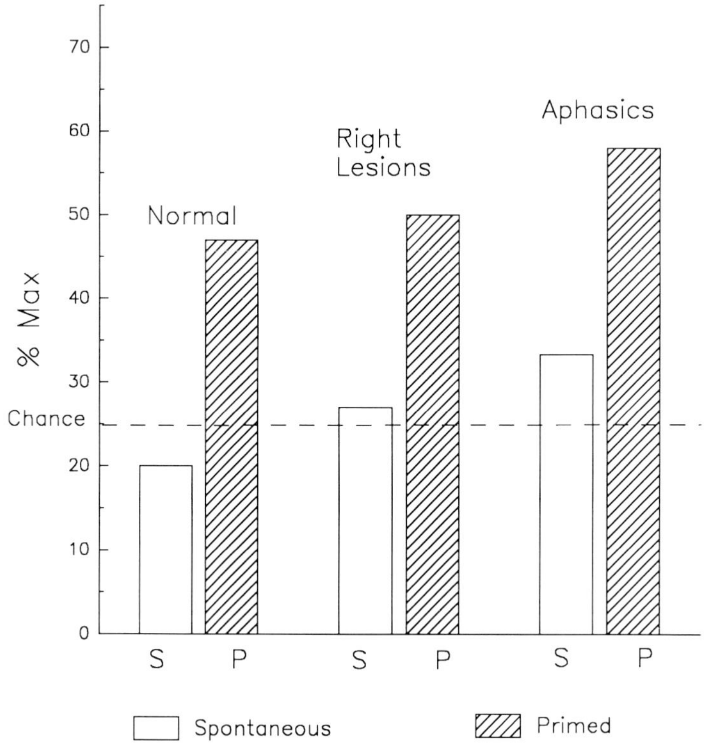

Fig. 11.6 Action/function choices on the Action/Function test.

either before or after priming (Fig. 11.6). Aphasic patients were, if anything, more likely than the other groups to make such a choice.

Alternative choices. The question arises whether the type of response, other than the target, differentiated the groups. After priming on Semantic categories, aphasic patients made fewer associative responses (Fig. 11.7), but this might have been a reciprocal of their higher number of semantic choices. However, on the Action/Function categories, where they did not differ from other groups, aphasics again made fewer associative choices than normals (Fig. 11.8). It appears, therefore, that severe aphasics are less likely than normals to make choices based on past temporal or spatial contiguity.

It appears from this study that globally aphasic patients are not only able to do semantic classifications, but do so more readily than normals or than patients with right-hemisphere pathology. Since the intact hemisphere in our extensively damaged aphasics is the right hemisphere, this may indicate that this hemisphere normally plays a leading

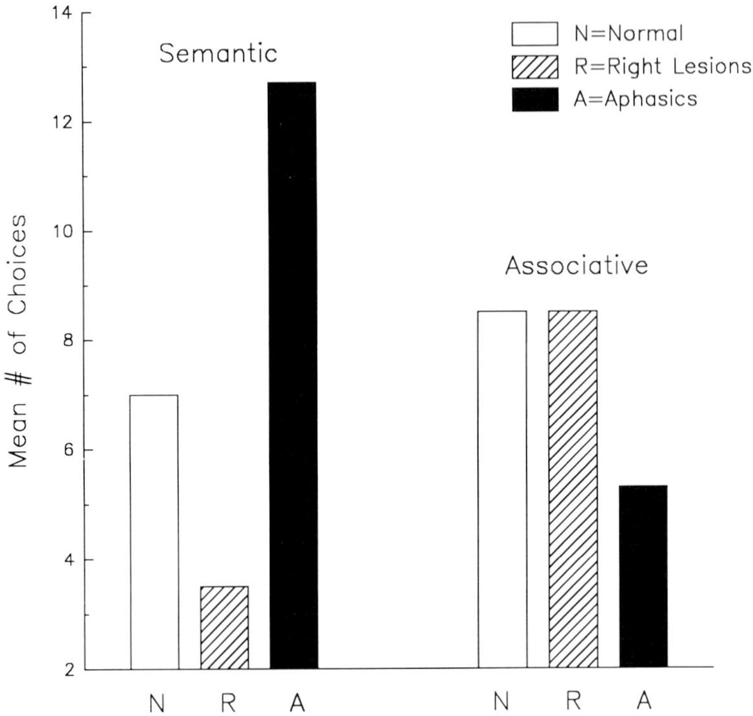

Fig. 11.7 Item choices after priming on Semantic Categories Task.

role in semantic categorization. This mode may become dominant when there is less or no interference from the left hemisphere, as in severe left-sided damage; whereas in normal persons, the intact left hemisphere may have a moderating effect on this tendency of the right hemisphere to operate via semantic categories. Alternatively, the intact left hemisphere in normal persons may permit the freer rein of associative solutions, or may substitute semantic categories of a more verbal nature. In any case, the findings are consistent with other studies suggesting a significant contribution to semantic processing from the right hemisphere (Zaidel, 1985; Joanette & coworkers, 1988).

Summary

Evidence is reviewed from various sources which suggests that the left hemisphere is not essential for semantic function, and that in fact the right hemisphere may play a leading role in nonlanguage semantic classification. The findings from the split-brain literature for semantic comprehension in the right hemisphere, the ability of "deep" dyslexics

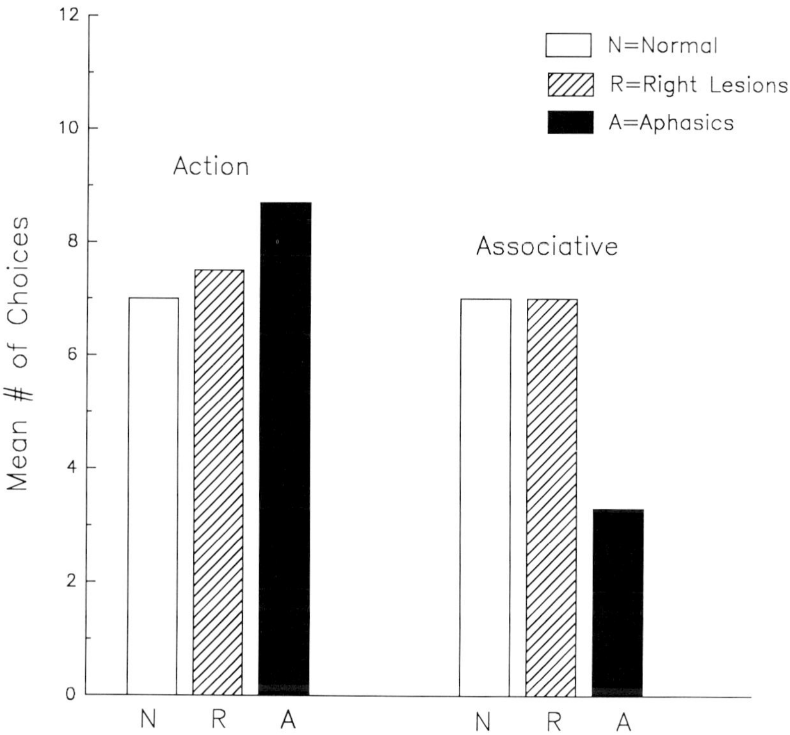

Fig. 11.8 Item choices after priming on Action/Function task.

to go from a letter array to the correct Semantic Category (albeit not necessarily the correct word), and the capacity of the great apes for semantic function in the absence of humantype language, all indicate that semanticity is not dependent on left-hemisphere language processing. Data from globally-aphasic patients suggest that semantic processing, as compared to associative linkage, may be favored by the right hemisphere.

Conclusion

The major conclusion from the data presented in this monograph is that the left cerebral hemisphere, in comparison with the right, is specialized for motor selection of both the oral and manual musculature. This is particularly true of movements specifiable within intrapersonal space, and it holds whether the movements to be programmed are components of a communication system or not. The parallels between communicative and noncommunicative movements are impressive. A consequent theme throughout is that human communication has been influenced by the characteristics of the motor programming systems control that the relevant oral and manual musculature. A manual system of communication may have preceded the vocal system we employ at present. This emphasis on the *behaviors* of speaking or of manual signing facilitates a comparative approach to the evolution of communication, emphasizing the continuity between humans and our primate relatives.

Most of the information we have on the neural basis of communication has come from studies of neurological patients with central nervous system disorders, especially disorders of speaking and of manual praxis. Such studies to date have usually consisted of compilations of individual cases with salient symptomatology, a methodology which not only omits negative cases but also tends to exaggerate functional dissociations. The neurological subjects of this monograph, in contrast, were selected solely on the basis of unilateral cerebral pathology, without reference to symptoms. They therefore represent an unbiased series of patients with lateralized brain lesions.

Lateralization of function in the brain is argued to be neither unique to humans nor specifically tied to the presence of complex language or other "higher level" functions. Asymmetry is a feature of many biological systems and neural lateralization may be secondary to other, possibly gonadal, asymmetries. We saw that, in humans, functional brain asymmetry for the control of speech production is present in the thalamus, basal ganglia, and cerebellum, not just in cerebral cortex. Moreover, it appears to be present for the most elementary of speech-control features, including voice volume and rhythm. The noncortical contributions to speech control do not merely mimic the function of the cortical regions with which they are connected, but show some distinctive characteristics.

Some findings were uncovered concerning the roles of the two major "cortical" speech areas in the left hemisphere, which would not be predicted from traditional aphasia typologies. Aphasic patients with damage restricted to the anterior or posterior speech zones, respectively, did not differ on various tasks of speech perception/comprehension. They did differ on measures of speech fluency, and on the type of speech-repetition task most affected. It appears that anterior and posterior speech systems represent two levels of speech control, unisyllabic and multisyllabic, respectively. Within the multisyllabic level, however, there are differences between temporal and parietal regions.

We have demonstrated a very tight association between the repetition of single syllables and reproduction of single nonspeech oral movements, and both were critically dependent on the left anterior region. Left posterior systems play a very minor role in controlling either speech or nonspeech single oral movements, but they do take part in selecting oral movements when more than one must be produced. Within the posterior region, the parietal system in many subjects is critical for the selection of articulatory/motor acts whether these involve speech or not. The temporal lobe, in contrast, appears to contribute a verbal-echolalic component.

Manual apraxia, a disturbance in making hand movements, is another common consequence of left-hemisphere pathology. This difficulty can occur quite independent of motor weakness, and typically manifests itself bilaterally. It appears to reflect the function of motor programming systems in frontal and parietal lobes, outside the Rolandic region. These praxis systems appear to be especially important for controlling movement within personal space, using the body as a framework. There is significant functional overlap between the manual praxis system and systems responsible for organizing multiple oral movements and speech.

Visuoconstructional disorders were also closely associated with manual apraxic difficulties, especially after left-sided damage. Constructionally apraxic patients with left-sided pathology showed the same repertoire of motor responses in handling manipulanda as did nonapraxic patients, but they emitted more of such movements in completing an act. This is consistent with the idea that their difficulties are related to limitations in selecting appropriate movements, rather than to motility or movement repertoire.

Disorders in manual sign language, which occur after pathology to the left hemisphere in right-handers, show characteristics similar to those of manual apraxia. Moreover, despite the highly visual nature of signing, comprehension of signs is affected by left cerebral damage rather than by right, even when right-hemisphere pathology results in gross left-sided neglect of space. This indicates that the processing of sign-language movements is not achieved by the systems representing external space. Moreover, the neuroanatomical areas affected in manual signing disorders appear to be the same as those affected in manual apraxia. It was suggested that manual sign aphasia may in fact be synonymous with manual apraxia, but that the apraxia in this instance is manifested also in linguistic categories of movement not usually available to hearing persons.

Consistent with previous literature, for patients who were not right-handed, speech representation was nevertheless found to be more dependent on the left hemisphere than on the right. Despite this, manual praxic function was more dependent on the right hemisphere. This was true for both ambidexters and left-handers. These findings raise some difficulty for explanations of left-handedness which propose that adextrality is simply the absence of dextrality. Our data suggest a lateralized manual programming mechanism that differentiates dextral and adextral persons.

Another individual difference that is associated with variation in functional brain organization is the sex of the subject. Sex differences in lateralization of function were shown for some fairly abstract verbal functions, such as vocabulary, which were more bilaterally organized in women, but not for basic speech function. No sex difference in degree of asymmetry was found for spatial rotation tasks, which were more dependent on the right hemisphere in both sexes. A much more compelling sex difference was uncovered, relating to *intra*hemispheric organization of function. For women, the anterior region in the left hemisphere appeared to be critical for speech and manual praxic function. The pattern in males showed a more even distribution of these functions across the two brain sectors, but in general favored the posterior region, particularly for manual control. For constructional tasks which also sample right-hemisphere function, anterior regions on the right were again more critical in women. These findings were related to the evolution of sexual dimorphism in human abilities, with males generally having better abilities relating to distance information and females to intra-personal space.

Finally, evidence was reviewed from various sources which suggested that the left hemisphere is not the hemisphere dominant for semantic function. Data collected on object classification in globally aphasic and right-damaged patients suggested that semantic processing, as compared to associative linkage, may be favored by the right hemisphere. These findings are compatible with the view that the left hemisphere's specialized functions are indeed related primarily to motor selection rather than to representational aspects of language.

References

Allen, L.S., Hines, M., Shryne, J.E., and Gorski, R.A. (1989). Two sexually dimorphic cell groups in the human brain. *Journal of Neuroscience,* **9**, 497–506.

Almgren, P.-E., Andersson, A.L., and Kullberg, G. (1969). Differences in verbally expressed cognition following left and right ventrolateral thalamotomy. *Scandinavian Journal of Psychology,* **10**, 243–9.

——, ——, and —— (1972). Long-term effects on verbally expressed cognition following left and right ventrolateral thalamotomy. *Confinia Neurologica,* **34**, 162–8.

Andrew, R.J. (1983). Lateralization of emotional and cognitive function in higher vertebrates, with special reference to the domestic chick. In *Advances in vertebrate neuroethology* (eds. J.P. Ewert, R.R. Capranica, and D.J. Ingle), NATO ASI series, Series A: *Life Sciences,* Vol. 56, pp. 477–509.

Annett, M. (1972). The distribution of manual asymmetry. *British Journal of Psychology,* **63**, 343–58.

Archibald, Y.M. (1987). Persisting apraxia in two left-handed aphasic patients with right-hemisphere lesions. *Brain & Cognition,* **6**, 412–28.

Arena, A. and Gainotti, G. (1978). Constructional apraxia and visuo-perceptive disabilities in relation to laterality of cerebral lesions. *Cortex,* **14**, 463–73.

Arendash, G.W. and Gorski, R.A. (1983). Effects of discrete lesions of the sexually dimorphic nucleus of the preoptic area or other medial preoptic regions on the sexual behavior of male rats. *Brain Research Bulletins,* **10**, 147–54.

Arrigoni, G. and deRenzi, E. (1964). Constructional apraxia and hemispheric locus of lesion. *Cortex,* **1**, 170–97.

Basso, A., Casati, G., and Vignolo, L.A. (1977). Phonemic identification defect in aphasia. *Cortex,* **13**, 84–95.

Bastian, H. and Lond, M.D. (1897). Some problems in connexion with aphasia and other speech defects. *Lancet,* **1**, 1187–1194.

Bates, E., Appelbaum, M., and Allard, L. (1991). Statistical constraints on the use of single cases in neuropsychological research. *Brain & Language,* **40**, 295–329.

Battison, R. (1974). Phonological deletion in American Sign Language. *Sign Language Studies,* **5**, 1–19.

—— (1978). *Lexical borrowing in American Sign Language.* Linstok Press, Silver Spring, MD.

—— and Padden, C. (1974). Sign language aphasia: a case study. Paper presented to the 49th meeting of the Linguistic Society of America, New York, December.

Bell, D.S. (1968). Speech functions of the thalamus inferred from the effects of thalamotomy. *Brain,* **91**, 619–38.

Benson, D.F. (1967). Fluency in aphasia: Correlation with radioactive scan localization. *Cortex,* **3**, 373–94.

Benton, A.L. (1972). The "minor" hemisphere. *Journal of the History of Medicine and Allied Sciences,* **27**, 5–14.

—— (1973). Visuoconstructive disability in patients with cerebral disease: its relationship to side of lesion and aphasic disorder. *Documenta Ophthalmologica,* **34**, 67–76.

—— and Hècaen, H. (1970). Stereoscopic vision in patients with unilateral cerebral disease. *Neurology,* **20**, 1084–8.

——, Hannay, H.J., and Varney, N.R. (1975). Visual perception of line direction in patients with unilateral brain disease. *Neurology,* **25**, 907–10.

——, Hamsher, de S.K., Varney, N.R., and Spreen, O. (1983). *Contributions to neuropsychological assessment.* Oxford University Press, New York.

Blumstein, S.E., Cooper, W.E., Zurif, E.B., and Caramazza, A. (1977). The perception and production of voice-onset time in aphasia. *Neuropsychologia,* **15**, 371–83.

Bogousslavsky, J., Van Melle, G., and Regli, F. (1988). The Lausanne stroke registry: analysis of 1000 consecutive patients with first stroke. *Stroke,* **19**, 1083–92.

Bonvillian, J.D., Orlansky, M.D., and Garland, J.B. (1982). Handedness patterns in deaf persons. *Brain and Cognition,* **1**, 141–57.

Brinkman, J. and Kuypers, H.G.J.M. (1973). Cerebral control of contralateral and ipsilateral arm, hand and finger movements in the split-brain rhesus monkey. *Brain,* **96**, 653–74.

Broca, P. (1960). Remarks on the seat of the faculty of articulate language, followed by an observaton of aphemia. In *The cerebral cortex* (G. von Bonin, ed. and trans.), pp. 49–72. Charles C. Thomas, Springfield. (Original published in 1861.)

Brodal, A. (1981). *Neurological anatomy*, p. 506. Oxford University Press, Oxford.

Brown, J.W. (1972). *Aphasia, apraxia and agnosia.* Charles C. Thomas, Springfield.

Bryden, M.P. (1982). *Laterality. Functional asymmetry in the intact brain.* Academic Press, New York.

Cain, D.P. and Wada, J.A. (1979). An anatomical asymmetry in the baboon brain. *Brain, Behavior and Evolution,* **16**, 222–6.

Cappa, S.F. and Vignolo, L.A. (1983). CT scan studies of aphasia. *Human Neurobiology,* **2**, 129–34.

—— and —— (1988). Sex differences in the site of brain lesions underlying global aphasia. *Aphasiology,* **2**, 259–64.

——, Papagno, C., Vallar, G., and Vignolo, L.A. (1986). Aphasia does not always follow left thalamic hemorrhage: a study of five negative cases. *Cortex,* **22**, 639–47.

Caramazza, A., Berndt, R.S., and Brownell, H.H. (1982). The semantic deficit hypothesis: perceptual parsing and object classification by aphasic patients. *Brain & Language,* **15**, 161–89.

Carmon, A. and Bechtoldt, H.P. (1969). Dominance of the right cerebral hemisphere for stereopsis. *Neuropsychologia,* **7**, 29–39.

Chapey, R. and Lubinski, R. (1979). Semantic judgment ability in adult aphasia. *Cortex,* **15**, 247–55.

Chiarello, C., Knight, R., and Mandel, M. (1982). Aphasia in a prelingually deaf woman. *Brain,* **105**, 29–51.

Ciemins, V.A. (1970). Localized thalamic hemorrhage. *Neurology,* **20**, 776–82.

Colombo, A., deRenzi, E., and Faglioni, P. (1976). The occurrence of visual neglect in patients with unilateral cerebral disease. *Cortex,* **12**, 221–31.

Coltheart, M. (1980). Deep dyslexia: a review of the syndrome. In *Deep dyslexia* (eds. M. Coltheart, K. Patterson, and J.C. Marshall), pp. 22–47. Routledge, London.

Conrad, K. (1949). Über aphasische Sprachstörungen bei hirnverletzten Linkshändern. *Nervenarzt,* **20**, 148–54.

Conrad, R. (1979). *The deaf schoolchild.* Harper & Row, London.

Corballis, M.C. and Beale, I.L. (1976). *The psychology of left and right.* Lawrence Erlbaum, Hillsdale, NJ.

Critchley, M. (1938). "Aphasia" in a partial deaf-mute. *Brain,* **61**, 163–9.

Crosby, E.C., Humphrey, T., and Lauer, E.W. (1962). *Correlative anatomy of the nervous system.* Macmillan, New York.

Damasio, H. and Damasio, A.R. (1980). The anatomical basis of conduction aphasia. *Brain,* **103**, 337–50.

—— and —— (1983). Localization of lesions in conduction aphasia. In *Localization in Neuropsychology* (ed. A. Kertesz), pp. 231–43. Academic Press, New York.

Darley, F.L., Aronson, A.E., and Brown, J.E. (1975). *Motor speech disorders. (Audio Seminars in Speech Pathology)* W.B. Saunders, Philadelphia.

Dejerine, J. (1913). Motor aphasia, anarthria, and apraxia. *Transactions of International Congress of Medicine,* 85–106.

deLacoste, M.C., Kirkpatrick, J.B., and Ross, E.D. (1985). Topography of the human corpus callosum. *Journal of Neuropathology and Experimental Neurology,* **44**, 578–91.

——, Holloway, R.L., and Woodward, D.J. (1986). Sex differences in the fetal human corpus callosum. *Human Neurobiology,* **5**, 93–6.

——, Horvath, D.S., and Woodward, D.J. (1988). Prosencephalic asymmetries in Lemuridae. *Brain. Behavior & Evolution,* **31**, 296–311.

——, ——, and —— (1991). Possible sex differences in the developing human fetal brain. *Journal of Clinical and Experimental Neuropsychology,* **13**, 831–46.

deLacoste-Utamsing, M.C. and Holloway, R.L. (1982). Sexual dimorphism in the human corpus callosum. *Science,* **216**, 1431–2.

deRenzi, E. and Vignolo, L.A. (1962). The Token test: a sensitive test to detect receptive disturbances in aphasics. *Brain,* **85**, 665–78.

—— and Faglioni, P. (1967). The relationship between visuo-spatial impairment and constructional apraxia. *Cortex,* **3**, 327–42.

——, Pieczuro, A., and Vignolo, L.A. (1966). Oral apraxia and aphasia. *Cortex,* **2**, 50–73.

——, ——, and —— (1968). Ideational apraxia: a quantitative study. *Neuropsychologia,* **6**, 41–52.

——, Faglioni, P., and Sorgato, P. (1982). Modality-specific and supramodal mechanisms of apraxia. *Brain,* **105**, 301–12.

Diamond, M.C., Dowling, G.A., and Johnson, R.E. (1981). Morphologic cerebral cortical asymmetry in male and female rats. *Experimental Neurology,* **71**, 261–8.

Douglass, E. and Richardson, J. (1959). Aphasia in a congenital deaf-mute. *Brain,* **82**, 68–80.

Ellis, A.W. and Young, A.W. (1988). *Human cognitive neuropsychology*. Lawrence Erlbaum, Hove (UK).

Ethelberg, S. (1951). Impairment of rapid complex movements and apraxia. *Acta Psychiatrica et Neurologica,* Supp. 75, 104–67.

Faglioni, P. and Basso, A. (1985). Historical perspectives on neuroanatomical correlates of limb apraxia. In *Neuropsychological studies of apraxia and related disorders* (ed. E.A. Roy), pp. 3–44. North-Holland/Elsevier, Amsterdam.

Falk, D. (1978). Cerebral asymmetry in Old World monkeys. *Acta Anatomica,* **101**, 334–9.

Faust, R. (1983). Selected aspects of spontaneous drawing in a group of unilaterally brain-damaged patients. Unpublished M.Sc. thesis, University of Waterloo, Waterloo, Ontario.

Fazio, C., Sacco, G., and Bugiani, O. (1973). The thalamic hemorrhage. *European Neurology,* **9**, 30–43.

Fischer, S.D. (1978). Sign language and creoles. In *Understanding language through sign language research* (ed. P. Siple), pp. 309–31. Academic Press, New York.

Fouts, R.S. (1973). Talking with chimpanzees. *Science Year,* 34–49.

Freud, S. (1891). *On aphasia.* [trans. E. Stengel]. International Universities Press, New York.

Gainotti, G. and Tiacci, C. (1970). Patterns of drawing disability in right and left hemispheric patients. *Neuropsychologia,* **8**, 379–84.

Gardner, B.T. and Gardner, R.A. (1971). Two-way communication with an infant chimpanzee. In *Behavior of nonhuman primates* (eds. A.M. Schrier and F. Stollnitz). Academic Press, New York.

Gardner, H. and Zurif, E. (1975). *Bee* but not *be*: oral reading of single words in aphasia and alexia. *Neuropsychologia,* **13**, 181–90.

Gardner, R.A. and Gardner, B.T. (1969). Teaching sign language to a chimpanzee. *Science,* **165**, 664–72.

Gazzaniga, M.S. (1963). Effects of commissurotomy on a preoperatively learned visual discrimination. *Experimental Neurology,* **8**, 14–19.

Gerendai, I. (1987). Laterality in the neuroendocrine system. In *Duality and unity of the brain* (ed. D. Ottoson), pp. 17–28. Wenner-Gren International Symposium Series, Vol. 47. Macmillan, London.

Geschwind, N. (1965). Disconnection syndromes in animals and man. Part II. *Brain,* **88**, 585–644.

—— (1967). The apraxias. In *Phenomenology of will and action* (eds. E.W. Straus and R.M. Griffith). Duquesne University.

—— (1972). Language and the brain. *Scientific American,* **226**, 76–83.

—— (1975). The apraxias: neural mechanisms of disorders of learned movement. *American Scientist,* **63**, 188–95.

—— (1979). Specializations of the human brain. *Scientific American,* **241**, 180–99.

—— and Levitsky, W. (1968). Human brain: left–right asymmetries in temporal speech region. *Science,* **161**, 186–7.

—— and Galaburda, A.M. (eds.) (1984). *Cerebral dominance: the biological foundations.* Harvard University Press, Cambridge.

Ghez, C. (1985). Voluntary movement. In *Principles of neural science* (eds. E. R. Kandel and J.H. Schwartz), pp. 487–501. Elsevier, New York.

Glass, A.V., Gazzaniga, M.S., and Premack, D. (1973). Artificial language training in global aphasics. *Neuropsychologia,* **11**, 95–103.

Gloning, I., Gloning, K., Haub, G., and Quatember, R. (1969). Comparison of verbal behavior in right-handed and non right-handed patients with anatomically verified lesion of one hemisphere. *Cortex*, **10**, 43–52.

Goodall, J. van Lawick (1971). *In the shadow of man.* Fontana Books, London.

Goodglass, H., Quadfasel, F.A., and Timberlake, W.H. (1964). Phrase length and the type and severity of aphasia. *Cortex,* **1**, 133–53.

Goy, R.W. and McEwen, B.S. (1980). *Sexual differentiation of the brain.* MIT Press, Cambridge, MA.

Graves, R. and Landis, T. (1985). Hemispheric control of speech expression in aphasia: a mouth asymmetry study. *Archives of Neurology,* **42**, 249–51.

——, Goodglass, H., and Landis, T. (1982). Mouth asymmetry during spontaneous speech. *Neuropsychologia,* **20**, 371–81.

Grober, E., Perecman, E., Kellar, L., and Brown, J. (1980). Lexical knowledge in anterior and posterior aphasics. *Brain & Language,* **10**, 318–30.

Groves, C.P. and Humphrey, N.K. (1973). Asymmetry in gorilla skulls: evidence of lateralized brain function? *Nature,* **244**, 53–4.

Guiot, G., Hertzog, E., Rondot, P., and Molina, P. (1961). Arrest or acceleration of speech evoked by thalamic stimulation in the course of stereotaxic procedures for Parkinsonism. *Brain,* **84**, 363–79.

Hamilton, C.R. and Vermeire, B.A. (1988*a*). Complementary hemispheric specialization in monkeys. *Science,* **242**, 1691–4.

—— and —— (1988*b*). Cognition, not handedness, is lateralized in monkeys. *Behavioral & Brain Sciences,* **11**, 723–5.

Hampson, E. and Kimura, D. (1992). Sex differences and hormonal influences on cognitive function in humans. In *Behavioral endocrinology* (eds. J. Becker, M. Breedlove and D. Crews) 357–98. MIT/Bradford Books, Cambridge.

Harris, L.J. (1980). Left-handedness: early theories, facts, and fancies. In *Neuropsychology of left-handedness* (ed. J. Herron), pp. 3–78. Academic Press, New York.

—— (1989). Footedness in parrots: three centuries of research, theory, and mere surmise. *Canadian Journal of Psychology,* **43**, 369–96.

Hayes, C. (1951). *The ape in our house.* Harper, New York.

Hècaen, H. (1962). Clinical symptomatology in right and left hemispheric lesions. In *Interhemispheric relations and cerebral dominance* (ed. V.B. Mountcastle), 215–43. Johns Hopkins, Baltimore.

—— and Consoli, S. (1973). Analyse des troubles du langage au cours des lésions de l'aire de Broca. *Neuropsychologia,* **11**, 377–88.

Heilman, K.M. (1973). Ideational apraxia—a re-definition. *Brain,* **96**, 861–4.

—— (1975). A tapping test in apraxia. *Cortex,* **11**, 259–63.

——, Rothi, L., and Kertesz, A. (1983). Localization of apraxia-producing lesions. In *Localization in Neuropsychology* (ed. A. Kertesz), pp. 371–92. Academic Press, New York.

Hermann, K., Turner, W.J., Gillingham, F.J., and Gaze, R.M. (1966). The effects of destructive lesions and stimulation of the basal ganglia on speech mechanisms. *Confinia Neurologica,* **27**, 197–207.

Hewes, G.W. (1973). Primate communication and the gestural origin of language. *Current Anthropology,* **14**, 5–32.

—— (1977). A model for language evolution. *Sign Language Studies,* **15**, 97–168.

Hines, M., Sloan, K., Lawrence, J., Lipcamon, J., and Chiu, L. (1988). The size of the human corpus callosum relates to language lateralization and to verbal ability. *Society for Neuroscience Abstracts,* **14**, No. 456.1.

Hockett, C.D. (1960). The origin of speech. *Scientific American,* **203**, 88–96.

Hollien, H. (1975). Neural control of the speech mechanism. In *The nervous system.* Vol. 3, *Human communication and its disorders* (ed. D.B. Tower), pp. 483–91. Raven, New York.

Holmes, G. (1922). The Croonian lectures on the clinical symptoms of cerebellar disease and their interpretations. In *Selected papers of Gordon Holmes* (ed. C.G. Phillips), pp. 186–247. Oxford University Press, Oxford (1979).

Inglis, J. and Lawson, J.S. (1981). Sex differences in the effects of unilateral brain damage on intelligence. *Science,* **212**, 693–5.

Ingram, D. (1975). Motor asymmetries in young children. *Neuropsychologia,* **13**, 95–102.

Jacobs, L.F., Gaulin, S.J.C., Sherry, D.F., and Hoffman, G.E. (1990). Evolution of spatial cognition: sex-specific patterns of spatial behavior predict hippocampal size. *Proceedings of the National Academy of Sciences,* **87**, 6349–52.

Joanette, Y. and Goulet, P. (1986). Criterion-specific reduction of verbal fluency in right brain-damaged right-handers. *Neuropsychologia,* **24**, 875–9.

——, ——, and LeDorze, G. (1988). Impaired word naming in right-brain-damaged right-handers: error types and time-course analysis. *Brain & Language,* **34**, 54–64.

Johanson, D. and Edey, M. (1981). *Lucy. The beginnings of mankind.* Warner Books, New York.

Jürgens, U. (1979). Neural control of vocalization in nonhuman primates. In *Neurobiology of social communication in primates* (eds. H.D. Steklis and M.J. Raleigh), pp. 11–44. Academic Press, New York.

—— (1989*a*). Primate communication: signaling, communication. In *Encyclopedia of Neuroscience* (ed. G. Adelman), Vol. 2, pp. 976–9. Birkhaüser, Boston.

—— (1989*b*). Cerebral analogues of speech mechanisms in non-human primates. Presented in session *Motor Control of Speech, International Neuropsychological Symposium, Dubrovnik.*

—— (1989*c*). Primate communication: signaling, vocalization. In *Speech and language* (ed. D. Kimura), pp. 11–13. Birkhäuser, Boston.

—— and vonCramon, D. (1982). On the role of the anterior cingulate cortex in phonation: a case report. *Brain & Language,* **15**, 234–48.

Katz, W.F. (1988). Anticipatory coarticulation in aphasia: acoustic and perceptual data. *Brain & Language,* **35**, 340–68.

Kellogg, W.N. (1968). Communication and language in the home-raised chimpanzee. *Science,* **162**, 423–7.

Kertesz, A. (1983). *Localization in Neuropsychology.* Academic Press, New York.

Kimura, D. (1961). Cerebral dominance and the perception of verbal stimuli. *Canadian Journal of Psychology,* **15**, 166–71.

—— (1963). Right temporal-lobe damage. Perception of unfamiliar stimuli after damage. *Archives of Neurology,* **8**, 264–71.

—— (1964). Left–right differences in the perception of melodies. *Quarterly Journal of Experimental Psychology,* **16**, 355–8.

—— (1966). Dual functional asymmetry of the brain in visual perception. *Neuropsychologia,* **4**, 275–85.

—— (1977). Acquisition of a motor skill after left-hemisphere damage. *Brain,* **100**, 527–42.

—— (1979). Neuromotor mechanisms in the evolution of human communication. In *Neurobiology of social communication in primates* (eds. H.D. Steklis and M.J. Raleigh), pp. 197–219. Academic Press, New York.

—— (1981). Neural mechanisms in manual signing. *Sign Language Studies,* **33**, 291–312.

—— (1982). Left-hemisphere control of oral and brachial movements and their relation to communication. *Philosophical Transactions of the Royal Society of London,* **B298**, 135–49.

—— (1983). Speech representation in an unbiassed sample of left-handers. *Human Neurobiology,* **2**, 147–54.

—— (1986). *Neuropsychology Test Procedures,* 108 pp. DK Consultants, London, Ontario.

—— (1987). Are men's and women's brains really different? *Canadian Psychology,* **28**, 133–47.

—— (1990). How special is language? Review of book by H. Poizner, E.S. Klima, and U. Bellugi entitled *What the hands reveal about the brain. Sign Language Studies,* **66**, 79–84.

—— (1992). Sex differences in the brain. *Scientific American,* September, **267**, 119–25.

—— and Vanderwolf, C.H. (1970). The relation between hand preference and the performance of individual finger movements by left and right hands. *Brain,* **93**, 769–74.

—— and Archibald, Y. (1974). Motor functions of the left hemisphere. *Brain,* **97**, 337–50.

—— and Durnford, M. (1974). Normal studies on the function of the right hemisphere in vision. In *Hemisphere function in the human brain* (eds. S.J. Diamond and J.G. Beaumont). Paul Elek, London.

—— and Davidson, W. (1975). Right arm superiority for tapping with distal and proximal joints. *Journal of Human Movement Studies,* **1**, 199–202.

—— and Humphrys, C.A. (1981). A comparison of left- and right-arm movements during speaking. *Neuropsychologia,* **19**, 807–12.

—— and Harshman, R.A. (1984). Sex differences in brain organization for verbal and nonverbal function. In *Sex differences in the brain (*eds. G.J. deVries *et al.*), pp. 423–41. *Progress in Brain Research*, Vol. 61. Elsevier, Amsterdam.

—— and Faust, R. (1987). Spontaneous drawing in an unselected sample of patients with unilateral cerebral damage. In *Duality and unity of the brain* (eds. D. Ottoson), pp. 114–46. Wenner-Gren Center International Symposium Series, Vol. 47. Macmillan.

—— and D'Amico, C. (1989). Evidence for subgroups of adextrals based on speech lateralization and cognitive patterns. *Neuropsychologia,* **27**, 977–86.

—— and Watson, N. (1989). The relation between oral movement control and speech. *Brain & Language,* **37**, 565–90.

—— and Hampson, E. (in press). Neural and hormonal mechanisms mediating sex differences in cognition. In *Biological approaches to the study of human intelligence.* (ed. P.A. Vernon), Ablex, Norwood, NJ.

——, Battison, R., and Lubert, B. (1976). Impairment of non-linguistic hand movements in a deaf aphasic. *Brain and Language,* **3**, 566–71.

——, Davidson, W., and McCormick, C.W. (1982). No impairment in sign language after right-hemisphere stroke. *Brain & Language,* **17**, 359–62.

——, Clydesdale, S., and Teasell, R. (1991). Semantic ability in aphasia. *Third IBRO World Congress of Neuroscience,* **3**, 178 (Abstract).

Klima, E.S. and Bellugi, U. (1979). *The signs of language.* Harvard University Press, Cambridge.

Kolb, B. (1990). Prefrontal cortex. In *The cerebral cortex of the rat* (eds. B. Kolb and R. Tees), 437–58. MIT Press, Cambridge.

—— and Whishaw, I.Q. (1990). *Fundamentals of human neuropsychology,* chapter 16. W.H. Freeman, New York.

Laitinen, L.V. and Vilkki, J. (1977). Observations on physiological and psychological functions of the ventral oral internal nucleus of the human thalamus. *Acta Neurologica Scandinavica,* **55**, 198–212.

Lansdell, H. (1961). The effect of neurosurgery on a test of proverbs. *American Psychologist,* **16**, 448 (Abstract).

—— (1962). A sex difference in effect of temporal-lobe neurosurgery on design preference. *Nature,* **194**, 852–4.

LaPointe, L.L. and Wertz, R.T. (1974). Oral-movement abilities and articulatory characteristics of brain-injured adults. *Perceptual and Motor Skills,* **39**, 39–46.

Leakey, M.D. (1979). *Olduvai Gorge.* Collins, London.

Lechtenberg, R. and Gilman, S. (1978). Speech disorders in cerebellar disease. *Annals of Neurology,* **3**, 285–90.

Lehmkuhl, G. and Poeck, K. (1981). A disturbance in the conceptual organization of actions in patients with ideational apraxia. *Cortex,* **17**, 153–8.

Leischner, A. (1943). Die "Aphasie" der Taubstummen. *Archiv. für Psychiatrie und Nervenkrankheiten,* **115**, 469–548.

Levy, J. and Trevarthen, C. (1977). Perceptual, semantic and phonetic aspects of elementary language processes in split-brain patients. *Brain,* **100**, 105–18.

—— and Levy, J.M. (1978). Human lateralization from head to foot: sex-related factors. *Science,* **200**, 1291–2.

Ley, R.G. and Bryden, M.P. (1982). A dissociation of right and left hemispheric effects for recognizing emotional tone and verbal content. *Brain & Cognition,* **1**, 3–9.

Liberman, A.M. (1982). On finding that speech is special. *American Psychologist,* **37**, 148–67.

Lichtheim, L. (1885). On aphasia. *Brain,* **7**, 433–84.

Lieberman, P. (1975). *On the origins of language: An introduction to the evolution of human speech.* Macmillan, New York.

Liepmann, H. (1908). *Drei Aufsätze aus dem Apraxiegebiet.* Karger Verlag, Berlin. [Trans. by D. Kimura (1980) as *Translations from Liepmann's essays on apraxia.* University of Western Ontario, Dept. Psychology Research Bulletin, No. 506.]

Marquardsen, J. (1969). The natural history of acute cerebrovascular disease. *Acta Neurologica Scandinavica,* **45** (Supp. 38), 7–188.

Marshall, J.C. and Newcombe, F. (1980). The conceptual status of deep dyslexia: an historical perspective. In *Deep dyslexia,* (eds. M. Coltheart, K. Patterson, and J.C. Marshall), pp. 1–21. Routledge, London.

Matarazzo, J.D. (1972). *Wechsler's Measurement and appraisal of adult intelligence.* Williams & Wilkins, Baltimore.

Mateer, C. (1978). Asymmetric effects of thalamic stimulation on rate of speech. *Neuropsychologia,* **16**, 497–9.

—— (1983). Motor and perceptual functions of the left hemisphere and their interaction. In *Language functions and brain organization* (ed. S.J. Segalowitz), pp. 145–70. Academic Press, New York.

—— and Kimura, D. (1977). Impairment of nonverbal oral movements in aphasia. *Brain and Language,* **4**, 153–83.

——, Polen, S.B., and Ojemann, G.A. (1982). Sexual variation in cortical localization of naming as determined by stimulation mapping. *Behavioral & Brain Sciences,* **5**, 310–11.

McFie, J., Piercy, M.F., and Zangwill, O.L. (1950). Visual–spatial agnosia associated with lesions of the right cerebral hemisphere. *Brain,* **73**, 167–90.

McGlone, J. (1980). Sex differences in human brain asymmetry: a critical survey. *Behavioral and Brain Sciences,* **3**, 215–63.

Menzel, E. W. (1973). Leadership and communication in young chimpanzees. In *Precultural primate behavior,* pp. 192–225. S. Karger, Basel.

Mettler, F.A. (1949). *Selective partial ablation of the frontal cortex,* pp. 74–6, 194–5, 370–89, 432–4, 449–52, 460–1. Paul Hoeber, New York.

Milner, B. and Kolb, B. (1985). Performance of complex arm and facial-movement sequences after cerebral commissurotomy. *Neuropsychologia,* **23**, 791–9.

Mittwoch, U. (1976). Lateral asymmetry and the function of the mammalian Y chromosome. In *Current Chromosome Research* (eds. K. Jones and P.E. Brandham), 195–201. Elsevier, Amsterdam.

—— (1985). Erroneous theories of sex determination. *Journal of Medical Genetics,* **22**, 164–70.

—— (1988). Ethnic differences in testis size: a possible link with the cytogenetics of true hermaphroditism. *Human Reproduction,* **3**, 445–9.

—— and Mahadevaiah, S. (1980). Additional growth—a link between mammalian testes, avian ovaries, gonadal asymmetry in hermaphrodites and the expression of H-Y antigen. *Growth,* **44**, 287–300.

Mizunuma, H., dePalatis, L.R., and McCann, S.M. (1983). Effect of unilateral orchidectomy on plasma FSH concentration; evidence for a direct neural connection between testes and CNS. *Neuroendocrinology,* **37**, 291–6.

Mohr, J.P. (1976). Broca's area and Broca's aphasia. In *Studies in neurolinguistics* (eds. H. Whitaker and H.A. Whitaker), pp. 201–35. Academic Press, New York.

——, Watters, W.C., and Duncan, G.W. (1975). Thalamic hemorrhage and aphasia. *Brain & Language,* **2**, 3–17.

Monrad-Krohn, G.H. (1947). Dysprosody or altered "melody of language." *Brain,* **70**, 405–15.

Moscovitch, M. (1979). Information processing and the cerebral hemispheres. In *Handbook of Behavioral Neurobiology* (Vol. 2, *Neuropsychology*) (ed. M.S. Gazzaniga). Plenum, New York.

Nathan, P.W. (1947). Facial apraxia and apraxic dysarthria. *Brain,* **70**, 449–78.

Nordeen, E.J. and Yahr, P. (1982). Hemispheric asymmetries in the behavioral and hormonal effects of sexually differentiating mammalian brain. *Science,* **218**, 391–4.

Nottebohm, F. (1981). Laterality, seasons and space govern the learning of a motor skill. *Trends in NeuroSciences,* 104–6.

—— (1987). Birdsong. *Encyclopedia of Neuroscience,* Vol. 1, pp. 133–6. Birkhäuser, Boston.

Ojemann, G.A. (1975). Language and the thalamus: object naming and recall during and after thalamic stimulation. *Brain & Language,* **2**, 101–20.

—— (1976). Subcortical language mechanisms. In *Studies in neurolinguistics, Vol. 1* (eds. H. Whitaker and H.A. Whitaker), pp. 103–38. Academic Press, New York.

—— (1977). Asymmetric function of the thalamus in man. *Annals of the New York Academy of Sciences,* **299**, 380–96.

—— (1983). Brain organization for language from the perspective of electrical stimulation mapping. *The Behavioral and Brain Sciences,* **6**, 189–230.

—— and Van Buren, J. (1967). Respiratory, heart rate and GSR responses from human diencephalon, *Archives of Neurology,* **16**, 74–8.

—— and Ward, A.A. (1973). Abnormal movement disorders. In *Neurological Surgery*, Vol. 3 (ed. J.R. Youmans), pp. 1829–67. W.B. Saunders, Philadelphia.

—— and Mateer, C. (1979). Human language cortex: Localization of memory, syntax, and sequential motor-phoneme identification systems. *Science,* **205**, 1401–3.

Paterson, A. and Zangwill, O.L. (1944). Disorders of visual space perception ciated with lesions of the right cerebral hemisphere. *Brain,* **67**, 331–58.

Patterson, F.G. (1978). The gestures of a gorilla: language acquisition in another pongid. *Brain & Language,* **5**, 72–97.

Penfield, W. and Roberts, L. (1959). *Speech and brain mechanisms.* Princeton University Press, Princeton.

Peterson, J.M. and Lansky, L.M. (1980). Success in architecture: handedness and/or visual thinking. *Perceptual & Motor Skills,* **50**, 1139–43.

Pieczuro, A. and Vignolo, L.A. (1967). Studio sperimentale sull'aprassia ideomotoria. *Sistema Nervoso,* **19**, 131–43.

Piercy, M., Hècaen, H., and Ajuriaguerra, J. de. (1960). Constructional apraxia associated with unilateral cerebral lesions—left and right sided cases compared. *Brain,* **83**, 225–42.

Poeck, H. (1969). Pathophysiology of emotional disorders associated with brain damage. In *Handbook of clinical neurology,* Vol. 3, *Disorders of higher nervous activity* (eds. P.J. Vinken and G.W. Bruyn), pp. 343–67. North-Holland, Amsterdam.

—— (1983). Ideational apraxia. *Journal of Neurology,* **230**, 1–5.

—— and Kerschensteiner, M. (1975). Analysis of the sequential motor events in oral apraxia. In *Cerebral localization* (eds. K.J. Zülch, O. Creutzfeldt, and G.C. Galbraith), pp. 98–111. Springer-Verlag, Berlin.

——, Lehmkuhl, G., and Willmes, K. (1982). Axial movements in ideomotor apraxia. *Journal of Neurology, Neurosurgery & Psychiatry,* **45**, 1125–9.

Poizner, H. and Battison, R. (1980). Cerebral asymmetry for sign language. In *Recent perspectives on American Sign Language.* (eds. H. Lane and F. Grosjean), pp. 79–101. Erlbaum, Hillsdale, NJ.

——, Klima, E.S., and Bellugi, U. (1987). *What the hands reveal about the brain.* MIT Press (Bradford), Cambridge.

Premack, D. (1971). Some general characteristics of a method for teaching language to organisms that do not ordinarily acquire it. In *Cognitive processes of nonhuman primates* (ed. L.E. Jarrard), pp. 47–82. Academic Press, New York.

Ramsay, D. (1980). Beginnings of bimanual handedness and speech in infants. *Infant Behavior & Development,* **3**, 67–77.

—— (1984). Onset of duplicated syllable babbling and unimanual handedness in infancy: evidence for developmental change in hemispheric specialization? *Developmental Psychology,* **20**, 64–71.

Rasmussen, T. and Milner, B. (1975). Clinical and surgical studies of the cerebral speech areas in man. In *Cerebral localization* (eds. K.J. Zülch, O. Creutzfeldt and G.C. Galbraith), pp. 238–55. Springer-Verlag, Berlin.

Richmond, G. and Clemens, L. (1988). Ventromedial hypothalamic lesions and cholinergic control of female sexual behavior. *Psychology and Behavior,* **42**, 179–82.

Riklan, M., Levita, E., Zimmerman, J., and Cooper, I.S. (1969). Thalamic correlates of language and speech. *Journal of Neurological Sciences,* **8**, 307–28.

Robinson, B.W. (1967). Vocalization evoked from forebrain in *Macaca mulatta. Psychology and Behavior,* **2**, 345–54.

Robinson, J.S. and Voneida, T.J. (1973). Hemisphere differences in cognitive capacity in the split-brain cat. *Experimental Neurology,* **38**, 123–34.

Rogers, L. (1989). The left and right of brains at work. *New Scientist,* 11 February, 56–9.

Ross, E.D. (1981). The aprosodias. *Archives of Neurology,* **38**, 561–69.

Rubens, A.B., Mahowald, M.W., and Hutton, J.T. (1976). Asymmetry of the lateral (Sylvian) fissures in man. *Neurology,* **26**, 620–4.

Russell, W.R. and Espir, M.L.E. (1961). *Traumatic aphasia.* University Press, Oxford.

Sanders, B., Soares, M.P., and D'Aquila, J.M. (1982). The sex difference on one test of spatial visualization: a nontrivial difference. *Child Development,* **53**, 1106–10.

Sarno, J., Swisher, L., and Sarno, M. (1969). Aphasia in a congenitally deaf man. *Cortex,* **5**, 398–414.

Sasanuma, S. (1980). Acquired dyslexia in Japanese: clinical features and underlying mechanisms. In *Deep dyslexia* (eds. M. Coltheart, K. Patterson, and J.C. Marshall), pp. 48–90. Routledge, London.

Schaltenbrand, G. (1965). The effects on speech and language of stereotactical stimulation in thalamus and corpus callosum. *Brain & Language,* **2**, 70–7.

Schuell, H. (1974). *Minnesota Test for Differential Diagnosis of Aphasia.* Univesity of Minnesota Press, Minneapolis.

Scoville, W.B. and Milner, B. (1957). Loss of recent memory after bilateral hippocampal lesions. *Journal of Neurology, Neurosurgery & Psychiatry,* **20**, 11–21.

Seidenberg, M.S. and Petitto, L. (1978). What do signing chimps have to say to linguists? *Chicago Linguistics Society,* **14**, 430–44.

Shallice, T. (1988). *From Neuropsychology to mental structure.* Cambridge University Press, New York.

Shankweiler, D. and Studdert-Kennedy, M. (1967). Identification of consonants and vowels presented to left and right ears. *Quarterly Journal of Experimental Psychology,* **19**, 59–63.

Sherry, D.F. and Vaccarino, A.L. (1989). Hippocampus and memory for food caches in black-capped chickadees. *Behavioral Neuroscience,* **103**, 308–18.

Shipley-Brown, F., Dingwall, W.O., Berlin, C.I., Yeni-Komshian, G.H., and Gordon-Salant, S. (1988). Hemispheric processing of affective and linguistic intonation contours in normal subjects. *Brain & Language,* **33**, 16–26.

Sperry, R. and Gazzaniga, M. (1967). Language following surgical disconnection of the hemispheres. In *Brain mechanisms underlying speech and language* (eds. C. Millikan and F. Darley), pp. 108–21. Grune & Stratton, New York.

Stewart, J. and Kolb, B. (1988). The effects of neonatal gonadectomy and prenatal stress on cortical thickness and asymmetry in rats. *Behavioral and Neural Biology,* **49**, 344–60.

Stokes, K. and Kimura, D. (1992). Stereoscopic function in patients with unilateral brain damage. Paper presented at the 3rd Annual Meeting of the Canadian Society for Brain, Behaviour, and Cognitive Science, Quebec City, June.

Stokoe, W.C. (1980). Sign language structure. *Annual Review of Anthropology,* **9**, 365–90.

——, Casterline, D.C., and Croneberg, C.G. (1965). (revised 1976). *A dictionary of American Sign Language on linguistic principles.* Linstok Press, Washington, DC.

Terrace, H.S. (1985). In the beginning was the "name." *American Psychologist,* **40**, 1011–28.

Tognola, G. and Vignolo, L.A. (1980). Brain lesions associated with oral apraxia in stroke patients: A clinico-neuroradiological investigation with the CT scan. *Neuropsychologia,* **18**, 257–72.

Tureen, L., Smolik, E., and Tritt, J. (1951). Aphasia in a deaf mute. *Neurology,* **1**, 237–44.

Umiker-Sebeok, D.J. and Sebeok, T.A. (eds.) (1978). *Aboriginal sign languages of the Americas and Australia.* Plenum Press, New York.

Van Buren, J.M. (1963). Confusion and disturbance of speech from stimulation in vicinity of the head of the caudate nucleus. *Journal of Neurosurgery,* **20**, 148–57.

Vignolo, L.A., Boccardi, E., and Caverni, L. (1986). Unexpected CT-scan findings in global aphasia. *Cortex,* **22**, 55–69.

von Monakow, C. (1914). *Die Localisation im Grosshirn.* J.F. Bergmann, Wiesbaden.

Wada, J.A., Clarke, R., and Hamm, A. (1975). Cerebral hemispheric asymmetry in humans. *Archives of Neurology,* **32**, 239–46.

Wallesch, C.-W., Kornhuber, H.H., Brunner, R.J., Kunz, T., Hollerbach, B., and Suger, G. (1983). Lesions of the basal ganglia, thalamus, and deep white matter: differential effects on language functions. *Brain & Language,* **20**, 286–304.

Warrington, E.K. (1969). Constructional apraxia. In *Handbook of clinical neurology*, Vol. 4 (eds. P.J. Vinken and G.W. Bruyn), pp. 67–83. North-Holland, Amsterdam.

—— and James, M.J. (1967). Disorders of visual perception in patients with localised cerebral lesions. *Neuropsychologia,* **5**, 253–66.

——, Logue, V., and Pratt, R.T.C. (1971). The anatomical localisation of selective impairment of auditory verbal short-term memory. *Neuropsychologia,* **9**, 377–87.

Watson, N.V. and Kimura, D. (1991). Nontrivial sex differences in throwing and intercepting: relation to psychometrically-defined spatial functions. *Personality & Individual Differences,* **12**, 375–85.

Webster, W.G. (1972). Functional asymmetry between the hemispheres of the cat. *Neuropsychologia,* **10**, 75–87.

—— (1981). Morphological asymmetries of the cat brain. *Brain, Behavior and Evolution,* **18**, 72–9.

Wechsler, D. (1955). *Wechsler Adult Intelligence Scale.* Psychological Corporation, New York.

—— (1958). *The measurement and appraisal of adult intelligence.* Williams & Wilkins, Baltimore.

—— (1981). *Wechsler Adult Intelligence Scale—Revised.* Psychological Corporation, New York.

Weisenburg, T. and McBride, K. (1935). *Aphasia.* Commonwealth Fund, New York.

Wernicke, C. (1874). *Der Aphasische Symptomencomplex.* Cohn & Weigert, Breslau.

—— (1911). The symptom-complex of aphasia. An authorized translation by J.L. Salinger. In *Diseases of the Nervous System* (ed. A. Church), pp. 265–324. Appleton, New York.

Wolf, M.E. and Goodale, M.A. (1987). Oral asymmetries during verbal and non-verbal movements of the mouth. *Neuropsychologia,* **25**, 375–96.

Woodward, J. (1978). Historical bases of American Sign Language. In *Understanding language through sign language research* (ed. P. Siple), pp. 333–48. Academic Press, New York.

Yeni-Komshian, G.H. and Benson, D.A. (1976). Anatomical study of cerebral asymmetry in the temporal lobe of humans, chimpanzees, and Rhesus monkeys. *Science,* **192**, 387–9.

Yerkes, R.M. and Learned, D.W. (1925). *Chimpanzee intelligence and its vocal expression.* Williams and Wilkes, New York.

Zaidel, D. and Sperry, R.W. (1977). Some long-term motor effects of cerebral commissurotomy in man. *Neuropsychologia,* **15**, 193–204.

Zaidel, E. (1978*a*). Lexical organization in the right hemisphere. In *Cerebral correlates of conscious experience* (eds. P. Buser and A. Rougeul-Buser). North-Holland, New York.

—— (1978*b*). Auditory language comprehension in the right hemisphere following cerebral commissurotomy and hemispherectomy: a comparison with child language and aphasia. In *Acquisition and language breakdown. Parallels and divergencies* (eds. A. Caramazza and E. Zurif), pp. 229–75. Johns Hopkins, Baltimore.

—— (1985). Language in the right hemisphere. In *The dual brain* (eds. D.F. Benson and E. Zaidel), pp. 205–31. Guilford, New York.

—— (1989). Language in the disconnected right hemisphere. In *Speech and language. Readings from the Encyclopedia of Neuroscience* (ed. D. Kimura), pp. 34–5. Birkhäuser, Boston.

Zangwill, O. (1975). Excision of Broca's area without persistent aphasia. In *Cerebral localization* (eds. K.J. Zülch, O. Creutzfeldt, and G.C. Galbraith), pp. 258–63. Springer-Verlag, Heidelberg.

—— (1960). Le problème de l'apraxie idéatoire. *Revue Neurologique,* **102**, 595–603.

Ziegler, W. and von Cramon, D. (1989). Die Sprachapraxie—eine apraktische Störung? *Fortschrift für Neurologie und Psychiatrie,* **57**, 198–204.

Author index

Subject index